The Big Plant B... Cookbook 2021

500+ Updated Recipes To Stay Healthy And Lose Weight On A Plant Based Diet

Heidi Page

TABLE OF CONTENTS

INTRODUCTION

A large number of individuals who have deliberately inspected creature agribusiness have made plans to go veggie lover. In any case, regardless of whether you choose a veggie lover diet isn't for you, you'll likely leave away from perusing this exposition sold on the advantages of eating what individuals currently call a "plant-based" diet. For what reason am I so sure? Since the motivations to pick an eating routine that is at any rate generally plant-based are overpowering to such an extent that there truly aren't any solid counterarguments. That may clarify why the most unmistakable nourishment governmental issues journalists—including Michael Pollan, Mark Bittman, and Eric Schlosser—advocate an eating routine dependent on plants.

Plant-based weight control plans convey a significant number of the advantages of being vegetarian while requiring just the scarcest exertion. Since you haven't dedicated yourself to being 100 percent anything, there's no motivation to stress that you'll cheat, slip, or mess up. You can follow a plant-based eating routine and still eat Thanksgiving turkey or a late spring grill. In the event that being 100 percent veggie lover is something individuals focus on, being plant-based is more something they incline toward.

Perhaps the best thing about the plant-based idea is that it frequently gets under way an "idealistic cycle," where one positive change prompts another and afterward to another. At the point when you normally attempt new veggie lover nourishments, your top picks will in general consequently become piece of your ordinary eating regimen. So as time passes by, your eating regimen will probably move in a veggie lover heading with no deliberate exertion on your part. A lot of current veggie lovers arrived by bit by bit sliding down the plant-based slant. After some time spent eating expanding measures of plant-based nourishments, they understood that they were only a couple of little and simple advances from turning out to be absolutely vegetarian.

There are various adorable and accommodating neologisms appended to the plant-based camp: reducetarian, flexitarian, chegan, plant-solid, and even veganish. On the off chance that any of these terms impacts you, simply snatch tightly to it and start thinking thusly as you start attempting more veggie lover and vegetarian suppers.

Also, there are a few other related ideas you may discover supportive, including:

Meatless Mondays, Mark Bittman's Vegan Before 6:00 arrangement, or taking a completely vegetarian diet out for a 21-day test drive. These conceivable outcomes can move huge change without forcing prerequisites for long lasting flawlessness.

Of the numerous motivations to go plant-based, maybe the best of all is the absence of a reasonable counterargument. In the entirety of my years expounding on nourishment legislative issues, I've not even once observed anybody (other than a couple paleo diet fan) make a genuine endeavor to contend against eating for the most part plants, since the preferences are unquestionable. Handfuls and many examinations show that eating more products of the soil can drastically diminish paces of malignant growth, diabetes, and circulatory malady. Furthermore, obviously, plant-based weight control plans likewise keep livestock from butcher, while all the while securing nature.

BREAKFAST & SMOOTHIES

01. Oatmeal & Peanut Butter Breakfast Bar

Preparation time: 10 minutes
Cooking Time 0 minutes
Servings 8

Ingredients

- 1½ cups date, pit removed
- ½ cup peanut butter
- ½ cup old-fashioned rolled oats

Directions:

1. Grease and line an 8" x 8" baking tin with parchment and pop to one side.
2. Grab your food processor, add the dates and whizz until chopped.
3. Add the peanut butter and the oats and pulse.
4. Scoop into the baking tin then pop into the fridge or freezer until set.
5. Serve and enjoy.

Nutrition:
Calories 459, Total Fat 8.9g, Saturated Fat 1.8g, Cholesterol 0mg, Sodium 77mg, Total Carbohydrate 98.5g, Dietary Fiber 11.3g, Total Sugars 79.1g, Protein 7.7g, Calcium 51mg, Potassium 926mg

02. Chocolate Chip Banana Pancake

Preparation time: 15 minutes
Cooking Time 3 minutes
Servings 6

Ingredients

- 1 large ripe banana, mashed
- 2 tablespoons coconut sugar
- 3 tablespoons coconut oil, melted
- 1 cup coconut milk
- 1 ½ cups whole wheat flour
- 1 teaspoon baking soda
- ½ cup vegan chocolate chips
- Olive oil, for frying

Directions:

1. Grab a large bowl and add the banana, sugar, oil and milk. Stir well.
2. Add the flour and baking soda and stir again until combined.
3. Add the chocolate chips and fold through then pop to one side.
4. Place a skillet over a medium heat and add a drop of oil.
5. Pour ¼ of the batter into the pan and move the pan to cover.
6. Cooking Time: for 3 minutes then flip and Cooking Time: on the other side.
7. Repeat with the remaining pancakes then serve and enjoy.

Nutrition:
Calories 315, Total Fat 18.2g, Saturated Fat 15.1g, Cholesterol 0mg, Sodium 221mg, Total Carbohydrate 35.2g, Dietary Fiber 2.6g, Total Sugars 8.2g, Protein 4.7g, Potassium 209mg

03. Avocado and 'Sausage' Breakfast Sandwich

Preparation time: 15 minutes
Cooking Time 2 minutes
Servings 1

Ingredients

- 1 vegan sausage patty
- 1 cup kale, chopped
- 2 teaspoons extra virgin olive oil
- 1 tablespoon pepitas
- Salt and pepper, to taste
- 1 tablespoon vegan mayo
- 1/8 teaspoon chipotle powder
- 1 teaspoon jalapeno chopped

- 1 English muffin, toasted
- ¼ avocado, sliced

Directions:

1. Place a sauté pan over a high heat and add a drop of oil.
2. Add the vegan patty and Cooking Time: for 2 minutes.
3. Flip the patty then add the kale and pepitas.
4. Season well then Cooking Time: for another few minutes until the patty is cooked.
5. Find a small bowl and add the mayo, chipotle powder and the jalapeno. Stir well to combine.
6. Place the muffin onto a flat surface, spread with the spicy may then top with the patty.
7. Add the sliced avocado then serve and enjoy.

Nutrition:

Calories 571, Total Fat 42.3g, Saturated Fat 10.1g, Cholesterol 36mg, Sodium 1334mg, Total Carbohydrate 38.6g, Dietary Fiber 6.6g, Total Sugars 3.7g, Protein 14.4g, Calcium 193mg

04. Black Bean Breakfast Burritos

Preparation time: 30 minutes
Cooking Time 10 minutes
Servings 4

Ingredients

- ¾ cup white rice
- 1 ½ cups water
- ¼ teaspoon sea salt
- ½ lime, juiced
- ¼ cup fresh cilantro, chopped
- 4 small red potatoes, cut into bite-sized pieces
- ½ red onion, sliced into rings
- 1-2 tablespoons olive oil
- Salt & pepper, to taste
- 1 cup cooked black beans
- ¼ teaspoon each ground cumin garlic powder, and chili powder
- Salt & pepper, to taste
- ¼ ripe avocado
- 1 lime, juiced
- 1 cup purple cabbage, thinly sliced
- 1 jalapeno, seeds removed, thinly sliced
- Pinch salt and black pepper
- 2 large vegan flour tortillas white or wheat
- ½ ripe avocado sliced
- ¼ cup salsa
- Hot sauce

Directions:

1. Place the rice, water and salt in a pan and bring to the boil.
2. Cover and Cooking Time: on low until fluffy then remove from the heat and pop to one side.
3. Place a skillet over a medium heat, add 1-2 tablespoons olive oil and add the potatoes and onion.
4. Season well then leave to Cooking Time: for 10 minutes, stirring often.
5. Remove from the heat and pop to one side.
6. Take a small pan then add the beans, cumin, garlic and chili. Stir well.
7. Pop over a medium heat and bring to simmer. Reduce the heat to keep warm.
8. Take a small bowl and add the avocado and lime. Mash together.
9. Add the cabbage and jalapeno and stir well. Season then pop to one side.
10. Grab the cooked rice and add the lime juice and cilantro then toss with a

fork.

11. Gently warm the tortillas in a microwave for 10-20 seconds then add the fillings.

12. Roll up, serve and enjoy.

Nutrition:

Calories 588, Total Fat 17.1g, Saturated Fat 3.4g, Sodium 272mg, Total Carbohydrate 94.8g, Dietary Fiber 16.2g, Total Sugars 5g, Protein 18.1g, Calcium 115mg, Iron 6mg, Potassium 1964mg

05. Cinnamon Rolls with Cashew Frosting

Preparation time: 30 minutes
Cooking Time 25 minutes
Servings 12

Ingredients

- 3 tablespoons vegan butter
- ¾ cup unsweetened almond milk
- ½ teaspoon salt
- 3 tablespoons caster sugar
- 1 teaspoon vanilla extract
- ½ cup pumpkin puree
- 3 cups all-purpose flour
- 2 ¼ teaspoons dried active yeast
- 3 tablespoons softened vegan butter
- 3 tablespoons brown sugar
- ½ teaspoon cinnamon
- ½ cup cashews, soaked 1 hour in boiling water
- ½ cup icing sugar
- 1 teaspoon vanilla extract
- 2/3 cup almond milk

Directions:

1. Grease a baking sheet and pop to one side.

2. Find a small bowl, add the butter and pop into the microwave to melt.

3. Add the sugar and stir well then set

aside to cool.

4. Grab a large bowl and add the flour, salt and yeast. Stir well to mix together.

5. Place the cooled butter into a jug, add the pumpkin puree, vanilla and almond milk. Stir well together.

6. Pour the wet ingredients into the dry and stir well to combine.

7. Tip onto a flat surface and knead for 5 minutes, adding extra flour as needed to avoid sticking.

8. Pop back into the bowl, cover with plastic wrap and pop into the fridge overnight.

9. Next morning, remove the dough from the fridge and punch down with your fingers.

10. Using a rolling pin, roll to form an 18" rectangle then spread with butter.

11. Find a small bowl and add the sugar and cinnamon. Mix well then sprinkle with the butter.

12. Roll the dough into a large sausage then slice into sections.

13. Place onto the greased baking sheet and leave in a dark place to rise for one hour.

14. Preheat the oven to 350°F.

15. Meanwhile, drain the cashews and add them to your blender. Whizz until smooth.

16. Add the sugar and the vanilla then whizz again.

17. Add the almond milk until it reaches your desired consistency.

18. Pop into the oven and bake for 20 minutes until golden.

19. Pour the glaze over the top then serve and enjoy.

Nutrition:

Calories 226, Total Fat 6.5g, Saturated Fat 3.4g, Cholesterol 0mg, Sodium 113mg, Total Carbohydrate 38g, Dietary Fiber 1.9g, Total Sugars 11.3g, Protein 4.9g, Calcium 34mg, Iron 2mg, Potassium 153mg

06. Sundried Tomato & Asparagus Quiche

Preparation time: 1 hour 20 minutes
Cooking Time 40 minutes
Servings 8

Ingredients

- 1 ½ cup all-purpose flour
- ½ teaspoon salt
- ½ cup vegan butter
- 2-3 tablespoons ice cold water
- 1 tablespoon coconut or vegetable oil
- ¼ cup white onion, minced
- 1 cup fresh asparagus, chopped
- 3 tablespoons dried tomatoes, chopped
- 1 x 14 oz. block medium/firm tofu, drained
- 3 tablespoons nutritional yeast
- 1 tablespoon non-dairy milk
- 1 tablespoon all-purpose flour
- 1 teaspoon dehydrated minced onion
- 2 teaspoons fresh lemon juice
- 1 teaspoon spicy mustard
- ½ teaspoon sea salt
- ½ teaspoon turmeric
- ½ teaspoon liquid smoke
- 3 tablespoons fresh basil, chopped
- 1/3 cup vegan mozzarella cheese
- Salt and pepper, to taste

Directions:

1. Preheat your oven to 350°F and grease 4 x 5" quiche pans and pop to one side.
2. Grab a medium bowl and add the flour and salt. Stir well.
3. Then cut the butter into chunks and add to the flour, rubbing into the flour with your fingers until it resembles breadcrumbs.
4. Add the water and roll together.
5. Roll out and place into the quiche pans.
6. Bake for 10 minutes then remove from the oven and pop to one side.
7. Place a skillet over a medium heat, add the oil and then add the onions.
8. Cooking Time: for five minutes until soft.
9. Throw in the asparagus and tomatoes and Cooking Time: for 5 more minutes. Remove from the heat and pop to one side.
10. Grab your food processor and add the tofu, nutritional yeast, milk, flour, onions, turmeric, liquid smoke, lemon juice and salt.
11. Whizz until smooth and pour into a bowl.
12. Add the asparagus mixture, the basil and the cheese and stir well.
13. Season with salt and pepper.
14. Spoon into the pie crusts and pop back into the oven for 15-20 minutes until set and cooked through.
15. Remove from the oven, leave to cool for 20 minutes then serve and enjoy.

Nutrition:

Calories 175, Total Fat 5.1g, Saturated Fat 2.3g, Cholesterol 1mg, Sodium 286mg, Total Carbohydrate 24.2g, Dietary Fiber 2.7g, Total Sugars 1.2g, Protein 9.4g, Calcium 118mg, Iron 3mg, Potassium 252mg

07. Gingerbread Waffles

Preparation time: 30minutes
Cooking Time 20 minutes
Servings 6

Ingredients

- 1 slightly heaping cup spelt flour
- 1 tablespoon ground flax seeds
- 2 teaspoons baking powder
- ¼ teaspoon baking soda
- ¼ teaspoon salt
- 1 ½ teaspoons ground cinnamon
- 2 teaspoons ground ginger
- 4 tablespoons coconut sugar
- 1 cup non-dairy milk
- 1 tablespoon apple cider vinegar
- 2 tablespoons black strap molasses
- 1½ tablespoons olive oil

Directions:

1. Find your waffle iron, oil generously and preheat.
2. Find a large bowl and add the dry ingredients. Stir well together.
3. Put the wet ingredients into another bowl and stir until combined.
4. Add the wet to dry then stir until combined.
5. Pour the mixture into the waffle iron and Cooking Time: on a medium temperature for 20 minutes
6. Open carefully and remove.
7. Serve and enjoy.

Nutrition:
Calories 256, Total Fat 14.2g, Saturated Fat 2g, Cholesterol 0mg, Sodium 175mg, Total Carbohydrate 31.2g, Dietary Fiber 3.4g, Total Sugars 13.2g, Protein 4.2g, Calcium 150mg, Iron 2mg, Potassium 369mg

08. Blueberry French Toast Breakfast Muffins

Preparation time: 55 minutes
Cooking Time 25 minutes
Servings 12

Ingredients

- 1 cup unsweetened plant milk
- 1 tablespoon ground flaxseed
- 1 tablespoon almond meal
- 1 tablespoon maple syrup
- 1 teaspoon vanilla extract
- 1 teaspoon cinnamon
- 2 teaspoons nutritional yeast
- ¾ cup frozen blueberries
- 9 slices soft bread
- ¼ cup oats
- 1/3 cup raw pecans
- ¼ cup coconut sugar
- 3 tablespoons coconut butter, at room temperature
- 1/8 teaspoon sea salt
- 9 slices bread, each cut into 4

Directions:

1. Preheat your oven to 375°F and grease a muffin tin. Pop to one side.
2. Find a medium bowl and add the flax, almond meal, nutritional yeast, maple syrup, milk, vanilla and cinnamon.
3. Mix well using a fork then pop into the fridge.
4. Grab your food processor and add the topping ingredients (except the coconut butter.Whizz to combine.
5. Add the butter then whizz again.
6. Grab your muffin tin and add a teaspoon of the flax and cinnamon batter to the bottom of each space.
7. Add a square of the bread then top with 5-6 blueberries.
8. Sprinkle with 2 teaspoons of the

crumble then top with another piece of bread.

9. Place 5-6 more blueberries over the bread, sprinkle with more of the topping then add the other piece of bread.

10. Add a tablespoon of the flax and cinnamon mixture over the top and add a couple of blueberries on the top.

11. Pop into the oven and Cooking Time: for 25-25 minutes until the top begins to brown.

12. Serve and enjoy.

Nutrition:

Calories 228, Total Fat 14.4g, Saturated Fat 5.1g, Cholesterol 0mg, Sodium 186mg, Total Carbohydrate 22.9g, Dietary Fiber 4g, Total Sugars 7.8g, Protein 4.3g, Calcium 87mg, Iron 2mg, Potassiuminutes

09. Greek Garbanzo Beans on Toast

Preparation time: 30 minutes
Cooking Time 5 minutes
Servings 2

Ingredients

- 2 tablespoons olive oil
- 3 small shallots, finely diced
- 2 large garlic cloves, finely diced
- ¼ teaspoon smoked paprika
- ½ teaspoon sweet paprika
- ½ teaspoon cinnamon
- ½ teaspoon salt
- ½-1 teaspoon sugar, to taste
- Black pepper, to taste
- 1 x 6 oz. can peel plum tomatoes
- 2 cups cooked garbanzo beans
- 4 slices of crusty bread, toasted
- Fresh parsley and dill
- Pitted Kalamata olives

Directions:

1. Pop a skillet over a medium heat and add the oil.
2. Add the shallots to the pan and Cooking Time: for five minutes until soft.
3. Add the garlic and Cooking Time: for another minute then add the other spices to the pan.
4. Stir well then add the tomatoes.
5. Turn down the heat and simmer on low until the sauce thickens.
6. Add the garbanzo beans and warm through.
7. Season with the sugar, salt and pepper then serve and enjoy.

Nutrition:

Calories 1296, Total Fat 47.4g, Saturated Fat 8.7g, Cholesterol 11mg, Sodium 1335mg, Total Carbohydrate 175.7g, Dietary Fiber 36.3g, Total Sugars 25.4g, Protein 49.8g, Calcium 313mg, Iron 17mg, Potassium 1972mg

10. Smoky Sweet Potato Tempeh Scramble

Preparation time: 17 minutes
Cooking Time 13 minutes
Servings 8

Ingredients

- 2 tablespoons olive oil
- 1 small sweet potato, finely diced
- 1 small onion, diced
- 2 garlic cloves, minced
- 8 oz. package tempeh, crumbled
- 1 small red bell pepper, diced
- 1 tablespoon soy sauce
- 1 tablespoon ground cumin
- 1 tablespoon smoked paprika
- 1 tablespoon maple syrup

- Juice of ½ lemon
- 1 avocado, sliced
- 2 scallions, chopped
- 4 tortillas
- 2 tbsp. Hot sauce

Directions:

1. Place a skillet over a medium heat and add the oil.
2. Add the sweet potato and Cooking Time: for five minutes until getting soft.
3. Add the onion and Cooking Time: for another five minutes until soft.
4. Stir through the garlic and Cooking Time: for a minute.
5. Add the tempeh, pepper, soy, cumin, paprika, maple and lemon juice and Cooking Time: for two more minutes.
6. Serve with the optional extras then enjoy.

Nutrition:
Calories 200, Total Fat 12.3g, Saturated Fat 2.2g, Cholesterol 0mg, Sodium 224mg, Total Carbohydrate 19g, Dietary Fiber 3.7g, Total Sugars 6.5g, Protein 7.5g, Calcium 64mg, Iron 2mg, Potassium 430mg

11. Fluffy Garbanzo Bean Omelet

Preparation time: 20 minutes
Cooking Time 7 minutes
Servings 2

Ingredients

- ¼ cup besan flour
- 1 tablespoon nutritional yeast
- ½ teaspoon baking powder
- ¼ teaspoon turmeric
- ½ teaspoon chopped chives
- ¼ teaspoon garlic powder
- 1/8 teaspoon black pepper
- ½ teaspoon Ener-G egg replacer

- ¼ cup water
- ½ cup Romaine Leafy Green Fresh Express
- ½ cup Veggies
- 1 tablespoon Salsa
- 1 tablespoon Ketchup
- 1 tablespoon Hot sauce
- 1 tablespoon Parsley

Directions:

1. Grab a medium bowl and combine all the ingredients except the greens and veggies. Leave to stand for five minutes.
2. Place a skillet over a medium heat and add the oil.
3. Pour the batter into the pan, spread and Cooking Time: for 3-5 minutes until the edges pull away from the pan.
4. Add the greens and the veggies of your choice then fold the omelet over.
5. Cooking Time: for 2 more minutes then pop onto a plate.
6. Serve with the topping of your choice.
7. Serve and enjoy.

Nutrition:
Calories 104, Total Fat 1.3g, Saturated Fat 0.2g, Cholesterol 0mg, Sodium 419mg, Total Carbohydrate 17.9g, Dietary Fiber 4.6g, Total Sugars 4.7g, Protein 6.6g, Calcium 69mg, Iron 3mg, Potassium 423mg

12. Easy Hummus Toast

Preparation time: 10 minutes
Cooking Time 0 minutes
Servings 1

Ingredients

- 2 slices sprouted wheat bread
- ¼ cup hummus
- 1 tablespoon hemp seeds

- 1 tablespoon roasted unsalted sunflower seeds

Directions:
1. Start by toasting your bread.
2. Top with the hummus and seeds then eat!

Nutrition:

Calories 445, Total Fat 16.3g, Saturated Fat 2.2g, Cholesterol 0mg, Sodium 597mg, Total Carbohydrate 54.5g, Dietary Fiber 10.5g, Total Sugars 6.1g, Protein 22.6g, Calcium 116mg, Iron 6mg, Potassium 471mg

13. No-Bake Chewy Granola Bars

Preparation time: 10 minutes
Cooking Time 10 minutes
Servings 8

Ingredients

- ¼ cup coconut oil
- ¼ cup honey or maple syrup
- ¼ teaspoon salt
- 1 teaspoon vanilla extract
- ½ teaspoon cardamominutes
- ¼ teaspoon cinnamon
- Pinch of nutmeg
- 1 cup old-fashioned oats
- ½ cup sliced raw almonds
- ¼ cup sunflower seeds
- ¼ cup pumpkin seeds
- 1 tablespoon chia seeds
- 1 cup chopped dried figs

Directions:
1. Line a 6" x 8" baking dish with parchment paper and pop to one side.
2. Grab a saucepan and add the oil, honey, salt and spices.
3. Pop over a medium heat and stir until it melts together.
4. Reduce the heat, add the oats and stir

to coat.
5. Add the seeds, nuts and dried fruit and stir through again.
6. Cooking Time: for 10 minutes.
7. Remove from the heat and transfer the oat mixture to the pan.
8. Press down until it's packed firm.
9. Leave to cool completely then cut into 8 bars.
10. Serve and enjoy.

Nutrition:

Calories 243, Total Fat 13.3g, Saturated Fat 6.7g, Cholesterol 0mg, Sodium 78mg, Total Carbohydrate 30.8g, Dietary Fiber 4.3g, Total Sugars 21.1g, Protein 4.2g, Calcium 67mg, Iron 2mg, Potassium 285mg

14. Hot Sausage and Pepper Breakfast Casserole

Preparation time: 57 minutes
Cooking Time 50 minutes
Servings 8

Ingredients

- 10 cup white bread, cubed
- 2¾ cups ice water
- 1 ¼ cup plant-based unsweetened creamer
- 2 tablespoons extra-virgin olive oil
- 3 vegan sausage, sliced
- 1 bell pepper, seeded and chopped
- 1 medium onion, chopped
- 2 garlic cloves, minced
- 5 cups spinach leaves
- 1 cup vegan parmesan, grated
- 1 teaspoon ground sea salt, or to taste
- ½ teaspoon ground nutmeg
- ½ teaspoon ground black pepper
- 1 tablespoon fresh parsley, chopped
- 1 teaspoon fresh rosemary, chopped
- 1 teaspoon fresh thyme, chopped

- 1 teaspoon fresh oregano, chopped
- 1 tablespoon vegan butter

Directions:

1. Preheat your oven to 375°F and grease a 13" x 8" baking dish.
2. Grab a medium bowl and add the water, milk and nutmeg. Whisk well until combined.
3. Pop a skillet over a medium heat and add the oil.
4. Add the sausage to the pan and Cooking Time: for 8-10 minutes until browned. Remove from the pan and pop to one side.
5. Add the onions and Cooking Time: for 3 minutes.
6. Add the peppers and Cooking Time: for 5 minutes.
7. Add the garlic, salt and pepper and Cooking Time: for 2 minutes then remove from the pan and pop to one side.
8. Add the spinach to the pan and Cooking Time: until wilted.
9. Remove the spinach from the pan then chop. Squeeze out the water.
10. Grab the greased baking dish and add half the cubed bread to the bottom.
11. Add half the spinach to the top followed by half the spinach and half of the onion and pepper mixture.
12. Sprinkle with half the parmesan then repeat.
13. Whisk the egg mixture again then pour over the casserole.
14. Pop into the oven and bake for 30 minutes until browned.
15. Serve and enjoy.

Nutrition:
Calories 263, Total Fat 8.2g, Saturated Fat 1g, Cholesterol 0mg, Sodium 673mg, Total Carbohydrate 31.8g, Dietary Fiber 3.4g, Total Sugars 3.6g, Protein 12.9g, Calcium 239mg, Iron 3mg, Potassium 377mg

15. Cardamom & Blueberry Oatmeal

Preparation time: 10 minutes
Cooking Time 3 minutes
Servings 1

Ingredients

- ¾ cup quick oats
- 1¼ cup water
- ½ cup unsweetened almond milk, divided
- 2 tablespoons pure maple syrup
- ¼ heaping teaspoon cinnamon
- 1/8 teaspoon cardamominutes
- Handful walnuts
- Handful dried currants

Directions:

1. Place the water into a small saucepan and bring to the boil.
2. Add the oats, stir through, reduce the heat to medium and Cooking Time: for 3 minutes.
3. Add half of the milk, stir again and Cooking Time: for another few seconds.
4. Remove from the heat and leave to stand for 3 minutes.
5. Transfer to a bowl and to with the remaining ingredients.
6. Drizzle with the milk then serve and enjoy.

Nutrition:
Calories 568, Total Fat 24.4g, Saturated Fat 1.9g, Cholesterol 0mg, Sodium 118mg, Total Carbohydrate 77g, Dietary Fiber 10.4g, Total Sugars 26.8g, Protein 16.5g, Vitamin D 1mcg, Calcium 263mg, Iron 5mg, Potassium 651mg

16. Cashew Cheese Spread

Preparation Time: 5 minutes
Cooking Time: 0 minutes
Servings: 5
Ingredients:

- 1 cup water
- 1 cup raw cashews
- 1 tsp. nutritional yeast
- ½ tsp. salt

Optional: 1 tsp. garlic powder
Directions:

1. Soak the cashews for 6 hours in water.
2. Drain and transfer the soaked cashews to a food processor.
3. Add 1 cup of water and all the other ingredients and blend.
4. For the best flavor, serve chilled.
5. Enjoy immediately, or store for later.

Nutrition:
Calories 162, Total Fat 12.7g, Saturated Fat 2.5g, Cholesterol 0mg, Sodium 239mg, Total Carbohydrate 9.7g, Dietary Fiber 1.1g, Total Sugars 1.5g, Protein 4.6g, Calcium 15mg, Iron 2mg, Potassium 178mg

17. Chilled Cantaloupe Smoothie

Preparation time: 10 minutes
Servings 2
Ingredients:

- 1½ cups cantaloupe, diced
- 2 Tbsp frozen orange juice concentrate
- ¼ cup white wine
- 2 ice cubes
- 1 Tbsp lemon juice
- ½ cup Mint leaves, for garnish

Directions:

1. Blend all ingredients to create a smooth mixture.

2. Top with mint leaves, and serve.

Nutrition:
Calories 349, Total Fat 13.1g, Saturated Fat 11.3g, Cholesterol 0mg, Sodium 104mg, Total Carbohydrate 50.5g, Dietary Fiber 5.5g, Total Sugars 46.4g, Protein 6.5g, Vitamin D 0mcg, Calcium 117mg, Iron 5mg, Potassium 1320mg

18. High Protein Peanut Butter Smoothie

Preparation time: 3 minutes
Servings: 2

Ingredients

- 2 cups kale
- 1 banana
- 2 tbsp. hemp seeds
- 1 tbsp. peanut butter
- 2/3 cup water
- 2 cups ice
- 1 cup almond or cashew milk
- 2 tbsp. cacao powder
- 1 scoop Vega vanilla protein powder

Directions:

1. Pop the kale and banana in a blender, then add the hemp seeds and peanut butter.
2. Add the milk, water and ice and blend until ingredients are combined.
3. Add the protein powder.
4. Pour into glasses and serve.

Nutrition:
Calories 687, Total Fat 50.4g, Saturated Fat 38g, Cholesterol 0mg, Sodium 176mg, Total Carbohydrate 46.5g, Dietary Fiber 9.9g, Total Sugars 23.7g, Protein 20.4g, Vitamin D 0mcg, Calcium 150mg, Iron 8mg, Potassium 979mg

19. Pineapple and Kale Smoothie

Preparation time: 3 minutes
Servings 2

Ingredients

- 1 cup Greek yogurt
- 1½ cups cubed pineapple
- 3 cups baby kale
- 1 cucumber
- 2 tbsp, hemp seeds

Directions:
1. Pop everything in a blender and blitz
2. Pour into glasses and serve.

Nutrition:
Calories 509, Total Fat 8.9g, Saturated Fat 3.3g, Cholesterol 10mg, Sodium 127mg, Total Carbohydrate 87.1g, Dietary Fiber 10.3g, Total Sugars 55.3g, Protein 30.6g, Vitamin D 0mcg, Calcium 438mg, Iron 5mg, Potassium 1068mg

20. Vanilla and Almond Smoothie

Preparation time: 3 minutes
Servings 1

Ingredients

- 2 scoops vegan vanilla protein powder
- ½ cup almonds
- 1 cup water

Directions:
1. Pop everything in a blender and blitz
2. Pour into glasses and serve.

Nutrition:
Calories 415, Total Fat 33.8g, Saturated Fat 1.8g, Cholesterol 0mg, Sodium 108mg, Total Carbohydrate 18.2g, Dietary Fiber 7.9g, Total Sugars 2g, Protein 42.1g, Vitamin D 0mcg, Calcium 255mg, Iron 9mg, Potassium 351mg

21. Berry Blast Smoothie

Preparation time: 3 minutes
Servings: 2

Ingredients

- 1 cup raspberries
- 1 cup frozen blueberries
- 1 cup frozen blackberries
- 1 cup almond milk
- ¼ cup Soy Yogurt

Directions:
1. Pop everything in a blender and blitz
2. Pour into glasses and serve.

Nutrition:
Calories 404, Total Fat 30.4g, Saturated Fat 25.5g, Cholesterol 0mg, Sodium 22mg, Total Carbohydrate 34.5g, Dietary Fiber 12.5g, Total Sugars 19.6g, Protein 6.3g, Vitamin D 0mcg, Calcium 112mg, Iron 4mg, Potassium 581mg

22. Choc-Banana Smoothie

Preparation time: 3 minutes
Servings: 2

Ingredients

- 1 banana
- 2 tbsp. hemp seeds
- 2/3 cup water
- 2 cups ice
- 1 cup almond or cashew milk
- 2 scoop Vegan chocolate protein powder
- 2 tbsp. cacao powder

Directions:
1. Pop everything in a blender and blitz
2. Pour into glasses and serve.

Nutrition:
Calories 676, Total Fat 52.3g, Saturated Fat 38.1g, Cholesterol 0mg, Sodium 46mg, Total Carbohydrate 41.6g, Dietary Fiber 8.7g, Total Sugars 25.2g, Protein 22.4g, Vitamin D 0mcg,

Calcium 80mg, Iron 6mg, Potassium 528mg

23. Greens and Berry Smoothie

Preparation time: 3 minutes
Servings 2

Ingredients

- 1 cup frozen berries
- 1 cup kale or spinach
- ¾ cup milk almond, oat or coconut milk
- ½ tbsp chia seeds

Directions:
1. Pop everything in a blender and blitz
2. Pour into glasses and serve.

Nutrition:
Calories 298, Saturated Fat 19.3g, Cholesterol 0mg, Sodium 29mg, Total Carbohydrate 20g, Dietary Fiber 7.4g, Total Sugars 8g, Protein 4.7g, Vitamin D 0mcg, Calcium 114mg, Iron 3mg, Potassium 520mg

24. Peanut Butter Banana Quinoa Bowl

Preparation time: 15 minutes
Cooking time: 15 minutes
Servings: 1
Ingredients:

- 175ml unsweetened soy milk
- 85g uncooked quinoa
- ½ teaspoon Ceylon cinnamon
- 10g chia seeds
- 30g organic peanut butter
- 30ml unsweetened almond milk
- 10g raw cocoa powder
- 5 drops liquid stevia
- 1 small banana, peeled, sliced

Directions:
1. In a saucepan, bring soy milk, quinoa, and Ceylon cinnamon to a boil.
2. Reduce heat and simmer 15 minutes.

3. Remove from the heat and stir in Chia seeds. Cover the saucepan with lid and place aside for 15 minutes.
4. In the meantime, microwave peanut butter and almond milk for 30 seconds on high. Remove and stir until runny. Repeat the process if needed.
5. Stir in raw cocoa powder and Stevia.
6. To serve; fluff the quinoa with fork and transfer in a bowl.
7. Top with sliced banana.
8. Drizzle the quinoa with peanut butter.
9. Serve.

Nutrition:
Calories 718
Total Fat 29.6g
Total Carbohydrate 90.3g
Dietary Fiber 17.5g
Total Sugars 14.5g
Protein 30.4g

25. Orange Pumpkin Pancakes

Preparation time: 10 minutes
Cooking time: 15 minutes
Servings: 4
Ingredients:

- 10g ground flax meal
- 45ml water
- 235ml unsweetened soy milk
- 15ml lemon juice
- 60g buckwheat flour
- 60g all-purpose flour
- 8g baking powder, aluminum-free
- 2 teaspoons finely grated orange zest
- 25g white chia seeds
- 120g organic pumpkin puree (or just bake the pumpkin and puree the flesh
- 30ml melted and cooled coconut oil
- 5ml vanilla paste

- 30ml pure maple syrup

Directions:

1. Combine ground flax meal with water in a small bowl. Place aside for 10 minutes.
2. Combine almond milk and cider vinegar in a medium bowl. Place aside for 5 minutes.
3. In a separate large bowl, combine buckwheat flour, all-purpose flour, baking powder, orange zest, and chia seeds.
4. Pour in almond milk, along with pumpkin puree, coconut oil, vanilla, and maple syrup.
5. Whisk together until you have a smooth batter.
6. Heat large non-stick skillet over medium-high heat. Brush the skillet gently with some coconut oil.
7. Pour 60ml of batter into skillet. Cooking Time: the pancake for 1 minute, or until bubbles appear on the surface.
8. Lift the pancake gently with a spatula and flip.
9. Cooking Time: 1 ½ minutes more. Slide the pancake onto a plate. Repeat with the remaining batter.
10. Serve warm.

Nutrition:
Calories 301
Total Fat 12.6g
Total Carbohydrate 41.7g
Dietary Fiber 7.2g
Total Sugars 9.9g
Protein 8.1g

26. Sweet Potato Slices With Fruits

Preparation time: 10 minutes
Cooking time: 10 minutes
Servings: 2

Ingredients:

The base:
- 1 sweet potato

Topping:
- 60g organic peanut butter
- 30ml pure maple syrup
- 4 dried apricots, sliced
- 30g fresh raspberries

Directions:

1. Peel and cut sweet potato into ½ cm thick slices.
2. Place the potato slices in a toaster on high for 5 minutes. Toast your sweet potatoes TWICE.
3. Arrange sweet potato slices onto a plate.
4. Spread the peanut butter over sweet potato slices.
5. Drizzle the maple syrup over the butter.
6. Top each slice with an equal amount of sliced apricots and raspberries.
7. Serve.

Nutrition:
Calories 300
Total Fat 16.9g
Total Carbohydrate 32.1g
Dietary Fiber 6.2g
Total Sugars 17.7g
Protein 10.3g

27. Breakfast Oat Brownies

Preparation time: 10 minutes
Cooking time: 40 minutes
Servings: 10 slices (2 per serving

Ingredients:
- 180g old-fashioned rolled oats
- 80g peanut flour
- 30g chickpea flour
- 25g flax seeds meal
- 5g baking powder, aluminum-free

- ½ teaspoon baking soda
- 5ml vanilla paste
- 460ml unsweetened vanilla soy milk
- 80g organic applesauce
- 55g organic pumpkin puree
- 45g organic peanut butter
- 5ml liquid stevia extract
- 25g slivered almonds

Directions:
1. Preheat oven to 180C/350F.
2. Line 18cm baking pan with parchment paper, leaving overhanging sides.
3. In a large bowl, combine oats, peanut flour, chickpea flour, flax seeds, baking powder, and baking soda.
4. In a separate bowl, whisk together vanilla paste, soy milk, applesauce. Pumpkin puree, peanut butter, and stevia.
5. Fold the liquid ingredients into dry ones and stir until incorporated.
6. Pour the batter into the prepared baking pan.
7. Sprinkle evenly with slivered almonds.
8. Bake the oat brownies for 40 minutes.
9. Remove from the oven and place aside to cool.
10. Slice and serve.

Nutrition:
Calories 309
Total Fat 15.3g
Total Carbohydrate 32.2g
Dietary Fiber 9.2g
Total Sugars 9.1g
Protein 13.7g

28. Spinach Tofu Scramble With Sour Cream

Preparation time: 10 minutes
Cooking time: 15 minutes
Servings: 2
Ingredients:
Sour cream:

- 75g raw cashews, soaked overnight
- 30ml lemon juice
- 5g nutritional yeast
- 60ml water
- 1 good pinch salt

Tofu scramble:

- 15ml olive oil
- 1 small onion, diced
- 1 clove garlic, minced
- 400 firm tofu, pressed, crumbled
- ½ teaspoon ground cumin
- ½ teaspoon curry powder
- ½ teaspoon turmeric
- 2 tomatoes, diced
- 30g baby spinach
- Salt, to taste

Directions:
1. Make the cashew sour cream; rinse and drain soaked cashews.
2. Place the cashews, lemon juice, nutritional yeast, water, and salt in a food processor.
3. Blend on high until smooth, for 5-6 minutes.
4. Transfer to a bowl and place aside.
5. Make the tofu scramble; heat olive oil in a skillet.
6. Add onion and Cooking Time: 5 minutes over medium-high.
7. Add garlic, and Cooking Time: stirring, for 1 minute.
8. Add crumbled tofu, and stir to coat with oil.

9. Add the cumin, curry, and turmeric. Cooking Time: the tofu for 2 minutes.
10. Add the tomatoes and Cooking Time: for 2 minutes.
11. Add spinach and cook, tossing until completely wilted, about 1 minute.
12. Transfer tofu scramble on the plate.
13. Top with a sour cream and serve.

Nutrition:
Calories 411
Total Fat 26.5g
Total Carbohydrate 23.1g
Dietary Fiber 5.9g
Total Sugars 6.3g
Protein 25g

29. Overnight Chia Oats

Preparation time: 15minutes + inactive time
Cooking time: 20 minutes
Servings: 4
Ingredients:
- 470ml full-fat soy milk
- 90g old-fashioned rolled oats
- 40g chia seeds
- 15ml pure maple syrup
- 25g crushed pistachios
- Blackberry Jam:
- 500g blackberries
- 45ml pure maple syrup
- 30ml water
- 45g chia seeds
- 15ml lemon juice

Directions:
1. Make the oats; in a large bowl, combine soy milk, oats, chia seeds, and maple syrup.
2. Cover and refrigerate overnight.
3. Make the jam; combine blackberries, maple syrup, and water in a saucepan.
4. Simmer over medium heat for 10 minutes.

5. Add the chia seeds and simmer the blackberries for 10 minutes.
6. Remove from heat and stir in lemon juice. Mash the blackberries with a fork and place aside to cool.
7. Assemble; divide the oatmeal among four serving bowls.
8. Top with each bowl blackberry jam.
9. Sprinkle with pistachios before serving.

Nutrition:
Calories 362
Total Fat 13.4g
Total Carbohydrate 52.6g
Dietary Fiber 17.4g
Total Sugars 24.6g
Protein 12.4g

30. Mexican Breakfast

Preparation time: 10 minutes
Cooking time: 10 minutes
Servings: 4
Ingredients:
- 170g cherry tomatoes, halved
- 1 small red onion, chopped
- 25ml lime juice
- 50ml olive oil
- 1 clove garlic, minced
- 1 teaspoon red chili flakes
- 1 teaspoon ground cumin
- 700g can black beans* (or cooked beans), rinsed
- 4 slices whole-grain bread
- 1 avocado, peeled, pitted
- Salt, to taste

Directions:
1. Combine tomatoes, onion, lime juice, and 15ml olive oil in a bowl.
2. Season to taste and place aside.
3. Heat 2 tablespoons olive oil in a skillet.

4. Add onion and Cooking Time: 4 minutes over medium-high heat.
5. Add garlic and Cooking Time: stirring for 1 minute.
6. Add red chili flakes and cumin. Cooking Time: for 30 seconds.
7. Add beans and Cooking Time: tossing gently for 2 minutes.
8. Stir in ¾ of the tomato mixture and season to taste.
9. Remove from heat.
10. Slice the avocado very thinly.
11. Spread the beans mixture over bread slices. Top with remaining tomato and sliced avocado.
12. Serve.

Nutrition:
Calories 476
Total Fat 21.9g
Total Carbohydrate 52.4g
Dietary Fiber 19.5g
Total Sugars 5.3g
Protein 17.1g

31. Amaranth Quinoa Porridge

Preparation time: 5 minutes
Cooking time: 35 minutes
Servings: 2
Ingredients:

- 85g quinoa
- 70g amaranth
- 460ml water
- 115ml unsweetened soy milk
- ½ teaspoon vanilla paste
- 15g almond butter
- 30ml pure maple syrup
- 10g raw pumpkin seeds
- 10g pomegranate seeds

Directions:
1. Combine quinoa, amaranth, and water.

2. Bring to a boil over medium-high heat.
3. Reduce heat and simmer the grains, stirring occasionally, for 20 minutes.
4. Stir in milk and maple syrup.
5. Simmer for 6-7 minutes. Remove from the heat and stir in vanilla, and almond butter.
6. Allow the mixture to stand for 5 minutes.
7. Divide the porridge between two bowls.
8. Top with pumpkin seeds and pomegranate seeds.
9. Serve.

Nutrition:
Calories 474
Total Fat 13.3g
Total Carbohydrate 73.2g
Dietary Fiber 8.9g
Total Sugars 10g
Protein 17.8g

32. Cacao Lentil Muffins

Preparation time: 10 minutes
Cooking time: 15 minutes
Servings: 12 muffins (2 per serving
Ingredients:

- 195g cooked red lentils
- 50ml melted coconut oil
- 45ml pure maple syrup
- 60ml unsweetened almond milk
- 60ml water
- 60g raw cocoa powder
- 120g whole-wheat flour
- 20g peanut flour
- 10g baking powder, aluminum-free
- 70g Vegan chocolate chips

Directions:
1. Preheat oven to 200C/400F.
2. Line 12-hole muffin tin with paper

cases.

3. Place the cooked red lentils in a food blender. Blend on high until smooth.
4. Transfer the lentils puree into a large bowl.
5. Stir in coconut oil, maple syrup, almond milk, and water.
6. In a separate bowl, whisk cocoa powder, whole-wheat flour, peanut flour, and baking powder.
7. Fold in liquid ingredients and stir until just combined.
8. Add chocolate chips and stir until incorporated.
9. Divide the batter among 12 paper cases.
10. Tap the muffin tin gently onto the kitchen counter to remove air.
11. Bake the muffins for 15 minutes.
12. Cool muffins on a wire rack.
13. Serve.

Nutrition:
Calories 372
Total Fat 13.5g
Total Carbohydrate 52.7g
Dietary Fiber 12.9g
Total Sugars 13g
Protein 13.7g

33. Chickpea Crepes With Mushrooms And Spinach

Preparation time: 20 minutes + inactive time
Cooking time: 15 minutes
Servings: 4
Ingredients:

Crepes:

- 140g chickpea flour
- 30g peanut flour
- 5g nutritional yeast
- 5g curry powder
- 350ml water
- Salt, to taste

Filling:

- 10ml olive oil
- 4 portabella mushroom caps, thinly sliced
- 1 onion, thinly sliced
- 30g baby spinach
- Salt, and pepper, to taste

Vegan mayo:

- 60ml aquafaba
- 1/8 teaspoon cream of tartar
- ¼ teaspoon dry mustard powder
- 15ml lemon juice
- 5ml raw cider vinegar
- 15ml maple syrup
- 170ml avocado oil
- Salt, to taste

Directions:

1. Make the mayo; combine aquafaba, cream of tartar, mustard powder. Lemon juice, cider vinegar, and maple syrup in a bowl.
2. Beat with a hand mixer for 30 seconds.
3. Set the mixer to the highest speed. Drizzle in avocado oil and beat for 10 minutes or until you have a mixture that resembles mayonnaise.
4. Of you want paler (in the color mayoadd more lemon juice.
5. Season with salt and refrigerate for 1 hour.
6. Make the crepes; combine chickpea flour, peanut flour, nutritional yeast, curry powder, water, and salt to taste in a food blender.
7. Blend until smooth.
8. Heat large non-stick skillet over medium-high heat. Spray the skillet with some cooking oil.
9. Pour ¼ cup of the batter into skillet

and with a swirl motion distribute batter all over the skillet bottom.

10. Cooking Time: the crepe for 1 minute per side. Slide the crepe onto a plate and keep warm.
11. Make the filling; heat olive oil in a skillet over medium-high heat.
12. Add mushrooms and onion and Cooking Time: for 6-8 minutes.
13. Add spinach and toss until wilted, for 1 minute.
14. Season with salt and pepper and transfer into a large bowl.
15. Fold in prepared vegan mayo.
16. Spread the prepared mixture over chickpea crepes. Fold gently and serve.

Nutrition:
Calories 428
Total Fat 13.3g
Total Carbohydrate 60.3g
Dietary Fiber 18.5g
Total Sugars 13.2g
Protein 22.6g

34. Goji Breakfast Bowl

Preparation time: 10 minutes
Servings: 2
Ingredients:
- 15g chia seeds
- 10g buckwheat
- 15g hemp seeds
- 20g Goji berries
- 235mml vanilla soy milk

Directions:
1. Combine chia, buckwheat, hemp seeds, and Goji berries in a bowl.
2. Heat soy milk in a saucepan until start to simmer.
3. Pour the milk over "cereals".
4. Allow the cereals to stand for 5 minutes.

5. Serve.

Nutrition:
Calories 339
Total Fat 14.3g
Total Carbohydrate 41.8g
Dietary Fiber 10.5g
Total Sugars 20g
Protein 13.1g

35. The 'Green Machine' Smoothie

Preparation time: 3 minutes
Servings 2

Ingredients
- 1 cup spinach
- ½ cup broccoli
- 2 Sticks of Celery
- 4 tbsp desiccated coconut
- 1 banana
- 1 scoop vegan unflavored protein powder
- 1 cup almond milk
- 1 cupwater

Directions:
1. Pop everything in a blender and blitz
2. Pour into glasses and serve.

Nutrition:
Calories 780, Total Fat 66.5g, Saturated Fat 57.9g, Cholesterol 0mg, Sodium 224mg, Total Carbohydrate 38.8g, Dietary Fiber 15g, Total Sugars 18.4g, Protein 19.6g, Vitamin D 0mcg, Calcium 82mg, Iron 5mg, Potassium 1108mg

36. Sweet Coffee and Cacao Smoothie

Preparation time: 3 minutes
Servings 2

Ingredients
- 2 tsp Coffee
- ½ a Banana

- 1 cup Almond Milk
- 1 tsp Cashew Butter
- 2 tsp Cacao Powder
- 1 tsp maple Syrup
- 1 scoop vegan protein powder
- ½ cup Chocolate

Directions:
1. Pop everything in a blender and blitz
2. Pour into glasses and serve.

Nutrition:
Calories 614, Total Fat 43.2g, Saturated Fat 34.6g, Cholesterol 10mg, Sodium 146mg, Total Carbohydrate 44.7g, Dietary Fiber 5.4g, Total Sugars 31.2g, Protein 17.6g, Vitamin D 0mcg, Calcium 104mg, Iron 4mg, Potassium 614mg

37. Amazing Blueberry Smoothie

Preparation time: 5 minutes
Servings 2
Ingredients:
- ½ avocado
- 1 cup frozen blueberries
- 1 cup raw spinach
- ¼ tsp sea salt
- 1 cup soy
- 1 frozen banana

Directions:
1. Blend everything in a powerful blender until you have a smooth, creamy shake.
2. Enjoy your healthy shake and start your morning on a fresh note!

Nutrition:
Calories 269, Total Fat 12.3g, Saturated Fat 2.3g, Cholesterol 0mg, Sodium 312mg, Total Carbohydrate 37.6g, Dietary Fiber 8.2g, Total Sugars 22.9g, Protein 6.4g, Vitamin D 0mcg, Calcium 52mg, Iron 3mg, Potassium 528mg

38. Go-Green Smoothie

Preparation time: 5 minutes
Servings 1
Ingredients:
- 2 tablespoons, natural cashew butter
- 1 ripe banana
- 2/3 cup, unsweetened coconut
- ½ cup kale

Directions:
1. Put everything inside a powerful blender.
2. Blend until you have a smooth, creamy shake.
3. Enjoy your special green smoothie.

Nutrition:
Calories 500, Total Fat 33.2g, Saturated Fat 18.9g, Cholesterol 0mg, Sodium 161mg, Total Carbohydrate 48.6g, Dietary Fiber 10.4g, Total Sugars 19.8g, Protein 9.1g, Vitamin D 0mcg, Calcium 72mg, Iron 9mg, Potassium 777mg

39. Creamy Chocolate Shake

Preparation time: 10 minutes
Servings 2
Ingredients:
- 2 frozen ripe bananas, chopped
- 1/3 cup frozen strawberries
- 2 tbsp cocoa powder
- 2 tbsp salted almond butter
- 2 cups unsweetened vanilla almond milk
- 1 dash Stevia or agave nectar
- 1/3 cup ice

Directions:
1. Add all ingredients in a blender and blend until smooth.
2. Take out and serve.

Nutrition:
Calories 272, Total Fat 14.3g, Saturated Fat

1.5g, Cholesterol 0mg, Sodium 315mg, Total Carbohydrate 37g, Dietary Fiber 7.3g, Total Sugars 16.8g, Protein 6.2g, Vitamin D 2mcg, Calcium 735mg, Iron 2mg, Potassium 732mg

40. Hidden Kale Smoothie

Preparation time: 5 minutes
Servings 2
Ingredients:

- 1 medium ripe banana, peeled and sliced
- ½ cup frozen mixed berries
- 1 tbsp hulled hemp seeds
- 2 cups frozen or fresh kale
- 2/3 cup 100% pomegranate juice
- 2¼ cups filtered water

Directions:

1. Add all ingredients in a blender and blend until smooth.
2. Take out and serve.

Nutrition:
Calories 164, Total Fat 2g, Saturated Fat 0.2g, Cholesterol 0mg, Sodium 51mg, Total Carbohydrate 34.2g, Dietary Fiber 3.9g, Total Sugars 17.7g, Protein 4.1g, Vitamin D 0mcg, Calcium 124mg, Iron 2mg, Potassium 776mg

41. Blueberry Protein Shake

Preparation time: 5 minutes
Servings 1
Ingredients:

- ½ cup cottage cheese
- 3 tbsp vanilla protein powder
- ½ cup frozen blueberries
- ½ tsp maple extract
- ¼ tsp vanilla extract
- 2 tsp flaxseed meal
- Sweetener, choice
- 10-15 ice cubes
- ¼ cup water

Directions:

1. Add all ingredients in a blender and blend until smooth.
2. Take out and serve.

Nutrition:
Calories 559, Total Fat 4.2g, Saturated Fat 1.9g, Cholesterol 14mg, Sodium 659mg, Total Carbohydrate 31.1g, Dietary Fiber 4.5g, Total Sugars 20.7g, Protein 98g, Vitamin D 0mcg, Calcium 518mg, Iron 3mg, Potassium 676mg

42. Raspberry Lime Smoothie

Preparation time: 5 minutes
Servings 2
Ingredients:

- 1 cup water
- 1 cup fresh or frozen raspberries
- 1 large frozen banana
- 2 tbsp fresh juice, lime
- 1 tsp oil, coconut
- 1 tsp agave

Directions:

1. In a blender put all ingredients and blend until smooth.
2. Take out and serve

Nutrition:
Calories 227, Total Fat 4g, Saturated Fat 1.3g, Cholesterol 0mg, Sodium 7mg, Total Carbohydrate 47.8g, Dietary Fiber 6g, Total Sugars 40.7g, Protein 0.9g, Vitamin D 0mcg, Calcium 22mg, Iron 1mg, Potassium 144mg

43. Peppermint Monster Smoothie

Preparation time: 5 minutes
Servings 1
Ingredients:

- 1 large frozen banana, peeled
- 1½ cups non-dairy milk
- A handful of fresh mint leaves, stems removed

- 1-2 handfuls spinach

Directions:
1. Add all ingredients in a blender and blend until smooth.
2. Take out and serve

Nutrition:
Calories 799, Total Fat 28.1g, Saturated Fat 16.7g, Cholesterol 110mg   , Sodium 645mg, Total Carbohydrate 98.4g, Dietary Fiber 4.5g, Total Sugars 77.2g, Protein 46.2g,   Vitamin D 7mcg, Calcium 1634mg, Iron 2mg, Potassium 1366mg

44. Banana Green Smoothie

Preparation time: 5 minutes
Servings 1
Ingredients:

- 1 cup coconut water
- ¾ cup plant-based milk
- ¼ tsp vanilla extract
- 1 heaping cup loosely packed spinach
- 2-3 cups frozen bananas, sliced

Directions:
Blend everything until smooth and serve.
Nutrition:
Calories 364, Total Fat 4.8g, Saturated Fat 2.6g, Cholesterol 15mg, Sodium 111mg, Total Carbohydrate 78g, Dietary Fiber 8g, Total Sugars 45.1g, Protein 9.6g, Vitamin D 1mcg, Calcium 257mg, Iron 1mg, Potassium 1241mg

45. Cinnamon Coffee Shake

Preparation time: 5 minutes
Servings 2
Ingredients:

- 1 cup cooled coffee, regular or decaf
- ¼ cup almond or non-dairy milk
- A few pinches cinnamon
- 2 tbsp hemp seeds
- Splash vanilla extract
- 2 frozen bananas, sliced into coins

- Handful of ice

Directions:
1. Chill some coffee in a sealed container for a couple of hours (or overnightbefore making this smoothie, or be ready to use more ice.
2. Add the non-dairy milk, cinnamon, vanilla, and hemp seeds to a blender and blend until smooth. Add the coffee and cut bananas and keep blending until smooth.
3. Add the ice and keep blending on high until there are no lumps remaining. Taste for sweetness and add your preferred plant-based sugar or sugar alternative.
4. Transfer to a glass and serve.

Nutrition:
Calories 197, Total Fat 6.4g, Saturated Fat 0.6g, Cholesterol 0mg, Sodium 5mg, Total Carbohydrate 31.3g, Dietary Fiber 5.2g, Total Sugars 15.8g, Protein 4g,   Vitamin D 0mcg, Calcium 53mg, Iron 1mg, Potassium 582mg

46. Orange Smoothie

Preparation time: 5 minutes
Servings 2
Ingredients:

- 1 cup orange slices
- 1 cup mango chunks
- 1 cup strawberries, chopped
- 1 cup coconut water
- Pinch freshly grated ginger
- 1-2 cups crushed ice

Directions:
Place everything in a blender, blend, and serve.
Nutrition:
Calories 269, Total Fat 12.3g, Saturated Fat 2.3g, Cholesterol 0mg, Sodium 312mg, Total

Carbohydrate 37.6g, Dietary Fiber 8.2g, Total Sugars 22.9g, Protein 6.4g, Vitamin D 0mcg, Calcium 52mg, Iron 3mg, Potassium 528mg

47. Pumpkin Smoothie

Preparation time: 5 minutes
Servings 2
Ingredients:

- 1 cup unsweetened non-dairy milk
- 2 medium bananas, peeled and cut into quarters and frozen
- 2 medjool dates, pitted
- 1 cup pumpkin puree, canned or fresh
- 2 cups ice cubes
- ¼ tsp cinnamon
- 2 tbsp ground flaxseeds
- 1 tsp pumpkin spice

Directions:
Blend all ingredients in a blender and serve.
Nutrition:
Calories 272, Total Fat 5.6g, Saturated Fat 2.2g, Cholesterol 10mg, Sodium 75mg, Total Carbohydrate 51.9g, Dietary Fiber 9.5g,Total Sugars 29.4g, Protein 8.2g, Vitamin D 1mcg, Calcium 204mg, Iron 4mg,Potassium 865mg

48. Turmeric Smoothie

Preparation time: 5 minutes
Servings 2
Ingredients:

- 2 cups non-dairy milk like coconut, almond
- 2 medium bananas, frozen
- 1 cup mango, frozen
- 1 tsp turmeric, ground grated, peeled
- 1 tsp fresh ginger, grated, peeled
- 1 tbsp chia seeds
- ¼ tsp vanilla extract
- ¼ tsp cinnamon, ground
- 1 pinch pepper, ground

Directions:
Blend all ingredients in a blender and serve
Nutrition:
Calories 785, Total Fat 62.4g, Saturated Fat 51.5g, Cholesterol 0mg, Sodium 41mg, Total Carbohydrate 60.2g, Dietary Fiber 15g, Total Sugars 33.9g, Protein 10g, Vitamin D 0mcg, Calcium 149mg, Iron 6mg, Potassium 1292mg

49. Veggie Smoothie

Preparation time: 10 minutes
Servings 1
Ingredients:

- 1 stalk celery
- 1 carrot peeled and roughly chopped
- ½ cup broccoli sprouts
- 1 cup kale, chopped
- ½ cup curly parsley
- ½ tomato roughly chopped
- ½ avocado
- 1 banana
- ½ green apple
- ½ cup non-dairy milk
- 1 tbsp chia seeds
- 1 tbsp flaxseeds

Directions:

1. Place all ingredients in a blender.
2. Blend until smooth. Serve immediately.

Nutrition:
Calories 696, Total Fat 34.1g, Saturated Fat 7g, Cholesterol 10mg, Sodium 190mg, Total Carbohydrate 90.5g, Dietary Fiber 29.5g, Total Sugars 37.2g, Protein 18.5g, Vitamin D 1mcg, Calcium 527mg, Iron 9mg, Potassium 2223mg

50. Very Berry Smoothie

Preparation time: 5 minutes
Servings 2
Ingredients:

- 2 cups, plant-based Milk
- 2 cups, Frozen or fresh berries
- ½ cup Frozen ripe bananas
- 2 teaspoons, Flax Seeds
- ¼ tsp, Vanilla
- ¼ tsp, Cinnamon

Directions:

1. Mix together milk, flax seeds, and fruit. Blend in a high-power blender.
2. Add cinnamon and vanilla. Blend until smooth.
3. Serve and enjoy!

Nutrition:

Calories 269, Total Fat 12.3g, Saturated Fat 2.3g, Cholesterol 0mg, Sodium 312mg, Total Carbohydrate 37.6g, Dietary Fiber 8.2g, Total Sugars 22.9g, Protein 6.4g, Vitamin D 0mcg, Calcium 52mg, Iron 3mg, Potassium 528mg

51. Coco Loco Smoothie

Preparation Time: 5 minutes
Servings: 2

Ingredients

- Coconut milk: 1 cup
- Frozen cauliflower florets: ½ cup
- Frozen mango cubes: 1 cup
- Almond butter: 1 tbsp

Directions:

1. Add all the ingredients to the blender
2. Blend on high speed to make it smooth

Nutrition:

Carbs: 18.2 g
Protein: 10.2 g
Fats: 27.0 g
Calories: 309 Kcal

52. Creamy Carrot Smoothie

Preparation Time: 5 minutes
Servings: 4

Ingredients

- Almond milk: 2 cups
- Prunes: 60 g
- Banana: 1
- Carrots: 150 g
- Walnuts: 30 g
- Ground cinnamon: ½ tsp
- Vanilla extract: 1 tsp
- Ground nutmeg: ¼ tsp

Directions:

1. Add all the ingredients to the blender
2. Blend on high speed to make it smooth

Nutrition:

Carbs: 14.9 g
Protein: 3 g
Fats: 4.5 g
Calories: 103 Kcal

53. Date Chocolate Smoothie

Preparation Time: 5 minutes
Servings: 2

Ingredients

- Unsweetened cocoa powder: 2 tbsp
- Unsweetened nut milk: 2 cups
- Almond butter: 2 tbsp
- Dried dates: 4 pitted
- Frozen bananas: 2 medium
- Ground cinnamon: ¼ tsp

Directions:

1. Add all the ingredients to the blender
2. Blend to form a smooth consistency

Nutrition:

Carbs: 72.1 g
Protein: 8 g
Fats: 12.7 g

Calories: 385 Kcal

54. Date Banana Pistachio Smoothie

Preparation Time: 5 minutes
Servings: 4

Ingredients

- Pistachios: 1 cup
- Raw pumpkin:175 g
- Cloves:1
- Nutmeg:1/8 tsp
- Dates: 4
- Banana:1
- Ground ginger:1/8 tsp
- Ground cinnamon:1 tsp
- Cashew milk:500 ml
- *Ice:* as per your need

Directions:
1. Add all the ingredients to the blender
2. Blend on high speed to make it smooth

Nutrition:
Carbs: 32.9 g
Protein: 9.7 g
Fats: 15 g
Calories: 320 Kcal

55. Fall Green Smoothie

Preparation Time: 5 minutes
Servings: 1

Ingredients

- Persimmon: 1
- Spinach: 1 cup
- Orange: 1
- Water: 1 cup
- Chia seeds:1 tbsp

Directions:
1. Add all the ingredients to the blender
2. Blend to form a smooth consistency
3. Add ice cubes from the top to chill it

Nutrition:
Carbs: 37.1 g
Protein: 6.5 g
Fats: 5.4 g
Calories: 183 Kcal

56. Fig Protein Smoothie

Preparation Time: 5 minutes
Servings: 1

Ingredients

- Fresh figs: 2
- Almond milk: 1 cup
- Dried date: 1 pitted
- Vanilla extract: ¼ tsp
- Sesame seeds: 2 tbsp

Directions:
1. Add all the ingredients to the blender
2. Blend to form a smooth consistency

Nutrition:
Carbs: 66.0 g
Protein: 16.1 g
Fats: 18 g
Calories: 435 Kcal

57. Frozen Berries Smoothie

Preparation Time: 5 minutes
Servings: 2

Ingredients

- Banana: 1 ripe
- Frozen berries: 200g
- Almond milk: 250ml

Directions:
1. Add all the ingredients in the blender
2. Blend to give a smooth consistency
3. Pour to the glasses and serve

Nutrition:
Carbs: 14.9 g
Protein: 2.2 g
Fats: 1.6 g
Calories: 92 Kcal

58. Fruit Medley Smoothie

Preparation Time: 5 minutes
Servings: 2

Ingredients

- Banana: 1 ripe sliced
- Almond milk: 1 cup
- Coconut oil: 1 tbsp
- Powdered ginger: 1 tsp
- Frozen fruit medley: 1 cup
- Chia seeds: 2 tbsp

Directions:

1. Add all the ingredients in the blender
2. Blend to give a smooth consistency
3. Pour to the glasses and serve

Nutrition:
Carbs: 52.8 g
Protein: 6.4 g
Fats: 22.5 g
Calories: 407 Kcal

59. Green Healthy Smoothie

Preparation Time: 5 minutes
Servings: 1

Ingredients

- Large banana: 1 frozen
- Fresh spinach: 1 cup
- Rolled oats: 2 tbsp
- Unsweetened almond milk: ¾ cup

Directions:

1. Add all the ingredients to the blender
2. Blend to form a smooth consistency

Nutrition:
Carbs: 41.2 g
Protein: 8.9 g
Fats: 3.9 g
Calories: 220 Kcal

60. Green Pina Colada

Preparation Time: 5 minutes
Servings: 2

Ingredients

- Full-fat coconut milk: 250 ml
- Fresh pineapple: 330 g chopped
- Banana: 1
- Fresh spinach: 30 g
- Water: 125 ml
- Sesame seeds: 2 tbsp

Directions:

1. Add all the ingredients to the blender
2. Blend to form a smooth consistency

Nutrition:
Carbs: 36.7 g
Protein: 6.4 g
Fats: 6.5 g
Calories: 198 Kcal

61. Guava Smoothie

Preparation Time: 5 minutes
Servings: 1

Ingredients

- Large banana: 1 frozen
- Guava: 2 cups deseeded and diced
- Unsweetened almond milk: ¾ cup

Directions:

1. Add all the ingredients to the blender
2. Blend to form a smooth consistency

Nutrition:
Carbs: 75g
Protein: 9.7 g
Fats: 3.6 g
Calories: 425Kcal

62. Halva Smoothie

Preparation Time: 5 minutes
Servings: 1

Ingredients

- Dried date: 1 pitted

- Tahini: 1 tbsp
- Fresh figs: 2
- Almond milk: 1 cup
- Vanilla extract: ¼ tsp

Directions:
1. Add all the ingredients to the blender
2. Blend to form a smooth consistency

Nutrition:
Carbs: 66.0 g
Protein: 12.1 g
Fats: 16.5g
Calories: 435 Kcal

63. Kale Smoothie

Preparation Time: 5 minutes
Servings: 1

Ingredients
- Almond butter: 1 tbsp
- Large banana: 1 frozen
- Fresh kale: 1 cup
- Unsweetened almond milk: ¾ cup

Directions:
1. Add all the ingredients to the blender
2. Blend to form a smooth consistency

Nutrition:
Carbs: 34.1
Protein: 12.8 g
Fats: 14 g
Calories: 244 Kcal

64. Kiwi And Almonds Smoothie

Preparation Time: 5 minutes
Servings: 2

Ingredients
- Almonds: ½ cup
- Coconut milk: 1 cup
- Kiwi: 1 medium peeled and sliced
- Banana:1 sliced
- Ice cubes: 4
- Avocado: 1/2 small

- Baby spinach:1 cup lightly packed

Directions:
1. Add all the ingredients to the blender
2. Blend to form a smooth consistency

Nutrition:
Carbs: 37.1 g
Protein: 15.2 g
Fats: 28.3 g
Calories: 427 Kcal

65. Mango Almonds Smoothie

Preparation Time: 5 minutes
Servings: 1

Ingredients
- Frozen mango chunks: 1 cup
- Almonds: ¼ cup whole
- Oat milk: ½ cup
- Frozen banana: 1 large sliced

Directions:
1. Add all the ingredients to the blender
2. Blend until smooth

Nutrition:
Carbs: 73.1 g
Protein: 10.5 g
Fats: 18.7 g
Calories: 486 Kcal

66. Mango Banana Smoothie

Preparation Time: 5 minutes
Servings: 1

Ingredients
- Almond butter: 1tbsp
- Frozen mango chunks: ½ cup
- Banana: 1 small
- Flax seeds: 1 tsp
- Ground cinnamon: ¼ tsp
- Hemp seeds: 1 tsp
- Coconut milk: 1 cup beverage

Directions:
1. Add all the ingredients to the blender

2. Blend to form a smooth consistency

Nutrition:

Carbs: 27.2 g

Protein: 10 g

Fats: 15.1 g

Calories: 270 Kcal

67. Orange Nuts Smoothie

Preparation Time: 5 minutes

Servings: 4 cups

Ingredients

- Peanuts: 1 cup
- Almonds: 1 cup
- Strawberries: 6
- Orange: 1
- Pineapple: 1 cup chopped
- Water: 1 cup

Directions:

1. Add all the ingredients to the blender
2. Blend to form a smooth consistency

Nutrition:

Carbs: 25.2 g

Protein: 15.5 g

Fats: 18.6 g

Calories: 462 Kcal

68. Peanut Butter Green Smoothie

Preparation Time: 5 minutes

Servings: 2

Ingredients

- Coconut milk: 1 cup
- Peanut butter: 2 tbsp
- Frozen banana: 1 small sliced
- Frozen zucchini: 1/2 cup sliced

Directions:

1. Add all the ingredients to the blender
2. Blend to form a smooth consistency

Nutrition:

Carbs: 33.1 g

Protein: 12.2 g

Fats: 18.0 g

Calories: 335 Kcal

69. Persimmon Mango Smoothie

Preparation Time: 5 minutes

Servings: 1

Ingredients

- Frozen mango chunks: ½ cup
- Carrot: 1 small peeled and chopped
- Coconut milk: 1 cup beverage
- Ground cinnamon: ¼ tsp
- Ripe persimmon: ½ ripe
- Flax seeds: 1 tsp
- Almond butter: 1tbsp
- Hemp seeds: 1 tsp

Directions:

1. Add all the ingredients to the blender
2. Blend to form a smooth consistency

Nutrition:

Carbs: 27.2 g

Protein: 10 g

Fats: 15.1 g

Calories: 256 Kcal

70. Pineapple, Orange, And Strawberry Smoothie

Preparation Time: 5 minutes

Servings: 4 cups

Ingredients

- Strawberries: 6
- Orange: 1
- Pineapple: 1 cup chopped
- Water: 1 cup

Directions:

1. Add all the ingredients to the blender
2. Blend to form a smooth consistency

Nutrition:

Carbs: 12.2 g

Protein: 2 g

Fats: 0.2 g

Calories: 48 Kcal

71. Pistachios Spinach Smoothie

Preparation Time: 5 minutes

Servings: 1

Ingredients

- Large banana: 1
- Ice cubes: 4
- Pistachios: ¼ cup
- Fresh spinach: 1 cup
- Rolled oats: 2 tbsp
- Unsweetened almond milk: ¾ cup

Directions:

1. Add all the ingredients to the blender
2. Blend to form a smooth consistency

Nutrition:

Carbs: 49.2 g

Protein: 12.9 g

Fats: 21.9 g

Calories: 392 Kcal

72. Peaches And Cream Oats

Servings: 2

Preparation time: 10 minutes

Cooking time: 3 minutes

Ingredients:

- 2 peaches, chopped
- 1 cup coconut milk
- 1 cup steel cut oats
- ½ vanilla bean
- 2 cups water

Directions:

1. Put the peaches in your instant pot.
2. Add coconut milk, oats, vanilla bean and water and Cooking Time: for 3 minutes.
3. Leave aside for 10 minutes to release

pressure and serve.

4. Enjoy!

Nutritional value: 130, fat 2, carbs 5, fiber 2, protein 3

73. Instant Pot Strawberries And Oats Breakfast

Servings: 2

Preparation time: 5 minutes

Cooking time: 10 minutes

Ingredients:

- 1/3 cup old-fashioned rolled oats
- 2 tablespoon dried strawberries
- A pinch of salt
- 2 cups water
- 2/3 cup almond milk
- ½ teaspoon coconut sugar

Directions:

1. Put the water in your instant pot.
2. Add strawberries, oats, almond milk and sugar.
3. Cooking Time: on High for 10 minutes, leave aside to release pressure, transfer the oats to breakfast bowls and serve.
4. Enjoy!

Nutritional value: calories 200, fat 5, carbs 25, fiber 2.8, protein 8.6

74. Instant Pot Breakfast Quinoa

Servings: 6

Preparation time: 10 minutes

Cooking time: 3 minutes

Ingredients:

- 1 and ½ cups quinoa
- 2 tablespoons maple syrup
- 2 and ¼ cups water
- ¼ teaspoon cinnamon, ground
- ½ teaspoon vanilla
- A pinch of salt

- Sliced almond for serving

Directions:
1. In your instant pot, mix water with maple syrup, quinoa, cinnamon, vanilla and salt.
2. Cooking Time: on high pressure for 1 minute, leave 10 minutes aside to release pressure, pour into breakfast bowls and serve with sliced almond on top.
3. Enjoy!

Nutritional value: 120, fat 10, carbs 12, fiber 4, protein 5

75. Carrot Breakfast

Servings: 6
Preparation time: 20 minutes
Cooking time: 10 minutes
Ingredients:
- 1 cup steel cut oats
- 4 cups water
- 1 tablespoon coconut butter
- 2 teaspoons cinnamon, ground
- 1 cup carrots, finely grated
- 3 tablespoons maple syrup
- 1 teaspoon pumpkin pie spice
- A pinch of salt
- ¼ cup chia seeds
- ¾ cup raisins

Directions:
1. In your instant pot, mix coconut butter with water, cinnamon, carrots, maple syrup, salt and pumpkin pie spice and Cooking Time: on High for 10 minutes.
2. Leave pot aside to release pressure for 10 minutes, add oats, chia seeds and raisins, cover pot and leave it aside for another 10 minutes.
3. Transfer the carrot oatmeal to breakfast bowls and serve it right

away!
4. Enjoy!

Nutritional value: calories 150, fat 3, carbs 12, sugar 13, fiber 8, protein 8

76. Special Instant Pot Vegan Pumpkin Oatmeal

Servings: 6
Preparation time: 10 minutes
Cooking time: 4 minutes
Ingredients:
- 1 and ½ cups steel cut oats
- 1 and ½ cups pumpkin puree
- 4 and ½ cups water
- 1 teaspoon allspice
- 1 teaspoon vanilla
- 2 teaspoons cinnamon powder
- ½ cup coconut sugar
- ¼ cup pecans, chopped
- 1 tablespoon cinnamon
- Almond milk for serving

Directions:
1. Put the water in your instant pot.
2. Add oats, pumpkin puree, 2 teaspoons cinnamon, vanilla and allspice.
3. Stir, cover, Cooking Time: on High for 3 minutes and then release pressure.
4. Meanwhile, in a bowl, mix pecans with sugar and 1 tablespoon cinnamon and stir well.
5. Sprinkle this over pumpkin oatmeal and serve with almond milk.
6. Enjoy!

Nutritional value: calories 130, fat 3, carbs 12, fiber 3, protein 4, sugar 10

77. Instant Pot Breakfast Risotto

Servings: 4
Preparation time: 10 minutes
Cooking time: 22 minutes
Ingredients:

- 1 and ½ cups arborio rice
- 2 apples, diced
- 2 tablespoons coconut butter
- A pinch of salt
- 1 and ½ teaspoons cinnamon
- 1/3 cup stevia
- 1 cup apple juice
- 3 cups almond milk
- ½ cup cherries, dried

Directions:

1. Put coconut butter and rice in your instant pot, cover and Cooking Time: on High for 6 minutes.
2. Uncover instant pot, stir the rice and mix it with apple juice, almond milk, apples, raw sugar, a pinch of salt and cinnamon, cover and Cooking Time: on High for 10 minutes.
3. Serve your breakfast rice in medium bowls with dried cherries on top.
4. Enjoy!

Nutritional value: calories 178, fat 12, carbs 1, fiber 3, protein 12, sugar 11

78. Instant Pot Breakfast Porridge

Servings: 6
Preparation time: 10 minutes
Cooking time: 35 minutes
Ingredients:

- ¼ cup split yellow gram, roasted
- 1 tablespoon split Bengal gram, roasted
- 1 and ½ cups banana, chopped
- 1 cup almond milk
- 1 cup rice, washed
- 3 cups water
- 2 cups jaggery, chopped
- 3 tablespoons cashews, chopped
- 1 teaspoon cardamom powder
- 2 tablespoons raisins
- ¼ teaspoon nutmeg powder
- Some saffron strands

Directions:

1. In your instant pot, mix yellow and Bengal gram with rice, almond milk and 2 and ½ cups water and Cooking Time: on High for 5-6 minutes.
2. Release pressure and leave aside for now.
3. In a bowl, mix jaggery with the rest of the water, stir and pour everything into a pan heated over medium high heat.
4. Cooking Time: for 7 minutes, stirring often and then add the rice and gram mix.
5. Stir again and Cooking Time: for 4 minutes.
6. Add raisins, cashews, stir and Cooking Time: for 2 minutes.
7. Add cardamom powder, nutmeg powder, saffron and bananas, stir and Cooking Time: for 1 minute.
8. Pour this into breakfast bowls and serve right away.
9. Enjoy!

Nutritional value: calories 70, fat 1, carbs 5, fiber 1, protein 1

79. Delicious Apple Butter

Servings: 80
Preparation time: 10 minutes
Cooking time: 1 hour
Ingredients:

- ½ cup cider vinegar
- 16 apples, cored and sliced
- 2 and ½ cups palm sugar
- ¼ teaspoon cloves, ground
- 3 teaspoons cinnamon

Directions:
1. Put the apples in your instant pot, cover and Cooking Time: on High for 1 hour.
2. Release pressure, transfer the apples to your food processor and blend them very well.
3. Return apples to your instant pot, add palm sugar, vinegar, cinnamon and cloves, stir well, cover the pot and Cooking Time: on Low for 15 minutes.
4. Transfer to jars and serve with some toasted bread in the morning.
5. Enjoy!

Nutritional value: calories 50, fat 0.1, carbs 11.2, fiber 0.9, sugar 10, protein 0.1

80. Instant Pot Vegan Chestnut Butter

Servings: 4
Preparation time: 10 minutes
Cooking time: 20 minutes
Ingredients:
- 1 and ½ pounds fresh chestnuts
- 11 ounces water
- 11 ounces coconut sugar

Directions:
1. Cut chestnuts in halves, peel them and put them in your instant pot.
2. Add water and sugar, cover lid and Cooking Time: on High for 20 minutes.
3. Release pressure for about 10 minutes, transfer the mix to your blender and pulse very well.

4. Pour into a bowl and serve in the morning on toasted and sliced bread.
5. Enjoy!

Nutritional value: calories 80, fat 0, carbs 20, sugar 17, protein 0

81. Delicious Breakfast Tapioca Pudding

Servings: 6
Preparation time: 10 minutes
Cooking time: 8 minutes
Ingredients:
- 1/3 cup tapioca pearls, washed and drained
- ½ cup water
- ½ cup coconut sugar
- 1 and ¼ cups almond milk
- Zest from ½ lemon

Directions:
1. Put the tapioca pearls in a bowl and mix with water, sugar, milk and lemon zest.
2. Stir well, transfer this to your instant pot and Cooking Time: on High for 8 minutes.
3. Release pressure, leave the pudding aside for 10 minutes, pour it into breakfast bowls and serve right away!
4. Enjoy!

Nutritional value: calories 180, fat 2.5, carbs 39, fiber 0.1, protein 2.5

82. Breakfast Quinoa Salad

Preparation time: 10 minutes
Cooking time: 20 minutes
Servings: 4
Ingredients:
- 1 yellow onion, chopped
- 3 tablespoons olive oil
- 1 carrot, chopped
- 2 cups mushrooms, sliced

- Zest from ½ lemon, grated
- 2 tablespoons lemon juice
- A pinch of salt and black pepper
- 4 garlic cloves, minced
- 1 cup quinoa
- 10 cherry tomatoes, halved
- 1 cup veggie stock
- 1 tablespoon spring onions, chopped

Directions:
1. Set your instant pot on sauté mode, add oil, heat it up, add onion and carrot, stir and sauté for 2 minutes.
2. Add mushrooms, stir and Cooking Time: for 3 minutes more.
3. Add salt, pepper, garlic, lemon juice and lemon zest, quinoa and stock, stir and Cooking Time: for 1 minute.
4. Add tomatoes, cover pot, Cooking Time: on High for 10 minutes, divide into bowls, sprinkle spring onion on top and serve cold for breakfast.
5. Enjoy!

Nutrition: calories 179, fat 2, fiber 3, carbs 18, protein 7

83. Cinnamon Oatmeal

Preparation time: 10 minutes
Cooking time: 4 minutes
Servings: 3
Ingredients:
- 3 cups water
- 1 cup steel cut oats
- 1 apple, cored and chopped
- 1 tablespoon cinnamon powder

Directions:
1. In your instant pot, mix water with oats, cinnamon and apple, stir, cover and Cooking Time: on High for 4 minutes.
2. Stir again, divide into bowls and serve for breakfast.

3. Enjoy!

Nutrition: calories 200, fat 1, fiber 7, carbs 12, protein 10

84. Breakfast Coconut Risotto

Preparation time: 10 minutes
Cooking time: 7 minutes
Servings: 4
Ingredients:
- 1 cup Arborio rice
- 2 cups almond milk
- 1 cup coconut milk
- 1/3 cup agave nectar
- 2 teaspoons vanilla extract
- ¼ cup coconut flakes, toasted

Directions:
1. Set your instant pot on simmer mode, add almond and coconut milk and bring to a boil.
2. Add agave nectar and rice, stir, cover and Cooking Time: on High for 5 minutes.
3. Add vanilla and coconut, stir, divide into bowls and serve warm.
4. Enjoy!

Nutrition: calories 192, fat 1, fiber 1, carbs 20, protein 4

85. Pumpkin Oats

Preparation time: 10 minutes
Cooking time: 3 minutes
Servings: 6
Ingredients:
- 4 and ½ cups water
- 1 and ½ cups steel cut oats
- 2 teaspoons cinnamon powder
- 1 teaspoon vanilla extract
- 1 teaspoon allspice
- 1 and ½ cup pumpkin puree
- ¼ cup pecans, chopped

Directions:

1. In your instant pot, mix water with oats, cinnamon, vanilla allspice and pumpkin puree, stir, cover and Cooking Time: on High for 3 minutes.
2. Divide into bowls, stir again, cool down and serve with pecans on top.
3. Enjoy!

Nutrition: calories 173, fat 1, fiber 5, carbs 20, protein 6

86. Simple Tofu Mix

Preparation time: 10 minutes
Cooking time: 10 minutes
Servings: 4
Ingredients:

- 1 pound extra firm tofu, cubed
- 1 cup sweet potato, chopped
- 3 garlic cloves, minced
- 2 tablespoons sesame seeds
- 1 yellow onion, chopped
- 2 teaspoons sesame seed oil
- 1 carrot, chopped
- 1 tablespoon tamari
- 1 tablespoon rice vinegar
- 2 cups snow peas, halved
- 1/3 cup veggie stock
- 2 tablespoons red pepper sauce
- 2 tablespoons scallions, chopped
- 2 tablespoons tahini paste

Directions:

1. Set your instant pot on sauté mode, add oil, heat it up, add sweet potato, onion and carrots, stir and Cooking Time: for 2 minutes.
2. Add garlic, half of the sesame seeds, tofu, vinegar, tamari and stock, stir and Cooking Time: for 2 minutes more.
3. Cover pot and Cooking Time: on High for 3 minutes more.
4. Add peas, the rest of the sesame seeds, green onions, tahini paste and pepper sauce, stir, cover and Cooking Time: on Low for 1 minutes more.
5. Divide into bowls and serve for breakfast.
6. Enjoy!

Nutrition: calories 172, fat 7, fiber 1, carbs 20, protein 6

87. Rich Quinoa Curry

Preparation time: 10 minutes
Cooking time: 12 minutes
Servings: 6
Ingredients:

- 1 sweet potato, chopped
- 1 broccoli head, florets separated
- 1 small yellow onion, chopped
- 15 ounces canned chickpeas, drained
- 28 ounces canned tomatoes, chopped
- 14 ounces coconut milk
- ¼ cup quinoa
- 1 tablespoon ginger, grated
- 2 garlic cloves, minced
- 1 tablespoon turmeric, ground
- 2 teaspoons tamari sauce
- 1 teaspoon chili flakes
- 1 teaspoon miso

Directions:

1. In your instant pot, mix potato with broccoli, onion, chickpeas, tomatoes, milk, quinoa, ginger, garlic, turmeric, tamari sauce, chili and miso, stir, cover and Cooking Time: on High for 12 minutes.
2. Stir one more time, divide into bowls and serve for breakfast.
3. Enjoy!

Nutrition: calories 400, fat 20, fiber 11, carbs 50, protein 12

88. Breakfast Burgers

Preparation time: 10 minutes
Cooking time: 30 minutes
Servings: 4
Ingredients:

- 1 cup mushrooms, chopped
- 2 teaspoons ginger, grated
- 1 cup yellow onion, chopped
- 1 cup red lentils
- 1 sweet potato, chopped
- 2 and ½ cups veggie stock
- ¼ cup hemp seeds
- ¼ cup parsley, chopped
- 1 tablespoon curry powder
- ¼ cup cilantro, chopped
- 1 cup quick oats
- 4 tablespoons rice flour

Directions:

1. Set your instant pot on sauté mode, add onion, mushrooms and ginger, stir and sauté for 2 minutes.
2. Add lentils, stock and sweet potatoes, stir, cover and Cooking Time: on High for 6 minutes.
3. Leave this mixture aside to cool down, mash using a potato masher, add parsley, hemp, curry powder, cilantro, oats and rice flour and stir well.
4. Shape 8 patties out of this mix, arrange them all on a lined baking sheet, introduce in the oven at 375 degrees F and bake for 10 minutes on each side.
5. Divide between plates and serve for breakfast.
6. Enjoy!

Nutrition: calories 140, fat 3, fiber 4, carbs 14, protein 13

89. Veggie Dumplings

Preparation time: 10 minutes
Cooking time: 15 minutes
Servings: 6
Ingredients:

- 1 tablespoon olive oil
- 1 cup mushrooms, chopped
- 1 and ½ cups cabbage, chopped
- ½ cup carrots, grated
- 1 and ½ cups water
- 2 tablespoons soy sauce
- 1 teaspoon ginger, grated
- 1 tablespoon rice wine vinegar
- 1 teaspoon sesame oil
- 12 vegan dumpling wrappers

Directions:

1. Set your instant pot on sauté mode, add olive oil, heat it up, add mushrooms, stir and Cooking Time: for 2 minutes.
2. Add carrot, cabbage, soy sauce and vinegar, stir and Cooking Time: for 3 minutes more.
3. Add sesame oil and ginger, stir and transfer everything to a bowl.
4. Arrange all wrappers on a working surface, divide veggie mix, wrap them and seal with some water.
5. Add the water to your instant pot, add steamer basket, add dumplings inside, cover pot and Cooking Time: on High for 7 minutes.
6. Divide between plates and serve for breakfast.
7. Enjoy!

Nutrition: calories 100, fat 2, fiber 1, carbs 9, protein 3

90. Breakfast Rice Bowl

Preparation time: 10 minutes
Cooking time: 30 minutes
Servings: 4
Ingredients:

- 1 tablespoon olive oil
- 2 tablespoons chana masala
- 1 red onion, chopped
- 1 tablespoon ginger, grated
- 1 tablespoon garlic, minced
- 1 cup chickpeas
- 3 cups water
- A pinch of salt and black pepper
- 14 ounces tomatoes, chopped
- 1 and ½ cups brown rice

Directions:

1. Set your instant pot on sauté mode, add the oil, heat it up, add onion, stir and Cooking Time: for 7 minutes.
2. Add salt, pepper, chana masala, ginger and garlic, stir and Cooking Time: for 1 minute more.
3. Add tomatoes, chickpeas, rice and water, stir, cover and Cooking Time: on High for 20 minutes.
4. Stir one more time, divide into bowls and serve for breakfast.
5. Enjoy!

Nutrition: calories 292, fat 4, fiber 3, carbs 9, protein 10

91. Millet And Veggie Mix

Preparation time: 10 minutes
Cooking time: 16 minutes
Servings: 4
Ingredients:

- 1 cup millet
- ½ cup oyster mushrooms, chopped
- 2 garlic cloves, minced
- ½ cup green lentils
- ½ cup bok choy, chopped
- 2 and ¼ cups veggie stock
- 1 cup yellow onion, chopped
- 1 cup asparagus, chopped
- 1 tablespoon lemon juice
- ¼ cup parsley and chives, chopped

Directions:

1. Set your instant pot on sauté mode, heat it up, add garlic, onion and mushrooms, stir and Cooking Time: for 2 minutes.
2. Add lentils and millet, stir and Cooking Time: for a few seconds more.
3. Add stock, stir, cover and Cooking Time: on High for 10 minutes.
4. Add asparagus and bok choy, stir, cover and leave everything aside for 3 minutes.
5. Add parsley and chives and lemon juice, stir, divide into bowls and serve for breakfast.
6. Enjoy!

Nutrition: calories 172, fat 3, fiber 8, carbs 19, protein 5

92. Tapioca Pudding

Preparation time: 10 minutes
Cooking time: 8 minutes
Servings: 4
Ingredients:

- 1/3 cup tapioca pearls
- ½ cup water
- 1 and ¼ cups almond milk
- ½ cup stevia
- Zest from ½ lemon, grated

Directions:

1. In a heatproof bowl, mix tapioca with almond milk, stevia and lemon zest and stir well.
2. Add the water to your instant pot, add

steamer basket, and heatproof bowl inside, cover and Cooking Time: on High for 8 minutes.

3. Stir your pudding and serve for breakfast.
4. Enjoy!

Nutrition: calories 187, fat 3, fiber 1, carbs 18, protein 3

93. Breakfast Arugula Salad

Preparation time: 10 minutes
Cooking time: 15 minutes
Servings: 6
Ingredients:

- 2 cups water
- 1 cup kamut grains, soaked for 12 hours, drained and mixed with some lemon juice
- 1 teaspoon sunflower oil
- A pinch of salt
- 4 ounces arugula
- 2 blood oranges, peeled and cut into medium segments
- 1 tablespoon olive oil
- 3 ounces walnuts, chopped

Directions:

1. In your instant pot, mix kamut grains with sunflower oil and the water, stir, cover and Cooking Time: on High for 15 minutes.
2. Drain kamut, transfer to a bowl, add a pinch of salt, arugula, orange segments, oil and walnuts, toss well and serve for breakfast.
3. Enjoy!

Nutrition: calories 125, fat 6, fiber 2, carbs 4, protein 3

94. Protein Blueberry Smoothie

Preparation Time: 5 minutes
Servings: 2

Ingredients

- Unsweetened coconut milk: 1 cup
- Blackberries: ½ cup
- Unsweetened coconut flakes: ¼ cup
- Banana: ½
- Chia Seeds Protein Powder: 2 scoops

Directions:

1. Add all the ingredients to the blender
2. Mix well and pour to the glass

Nutritional Facts

Carbs: 24.0 g
Protein: 23.1 g
Fats: 11.2 g
Calories: 376 Kcal

95. Pumpkin Pie Smoothie

Preparation Time: 5 minutes
Servings: 4

Ingredients

- Raw pumpkin:175 g
- Cloves:1
- Nutmeg:1/8 tsp
- Dates: 4
- Banana:1
- Ground ginger:1/8 tsp
- Ground cinnamon:1 tsp
- Cashew milk:500 ml
- Ice: as per your need

Directions:

1. Add all the ingredients to the blender
2. Blend on high speed to make it smooth

Nutrition:
Carbs: 24.9 g
Protein: 3.5 g
Fats: 1 g

Calories: 148 Kcal

96. Smoothie Bowl

Preparation Time: 5 minutes
Servings: 2

Ingredients

- Unsweetened almond milk: 250 ml
- Frozen Bananas: 2 large
- Peanut butter:2 tbsp
- Frozen blueberries:140 g
- Pistachios: 2 tbsp chopped

Directions:

1. Add all the ingredients to the blender except pistachios and blend well
2. Add fresh berries on top and pistachios and serve

Nutrition:
Carbs: 41.6 g
Protein: 7 g
Fats: 16.4 g
Calories: 261 Kcal

97. Soothing After Workout Smoothie

Preparation Time: 5 minutes
Servings: 2

Ingredients

- Strawberries: 1 cup chopped
- Oat milk: 1 cup
- Banana: 1
- Peanut butter: 1 tbsp

Directions:

1. Add all the ingredients to the blender
2. Blend on high speed to make it smooth

Nutrition:
Carbs: 26.7g
Protein: 7g
Fats: 8.5g
Calories: 198 Kcal

98. Strawberry Coconut Smoothie

Preparation Time: 5 minutes
Servings: 2

Ingredients

- Coconut milk: 1 cup
- Strawberry: 1 cup
- Almond butter: 1 tbsp
- Frozen mango cubes: ½ cup

Directions:

1. Add all the ingredients to the blender
2. Blend on high speed to make it smooth

Nutritional Facts
Carbs: 18.8 g
Protein: 8 g
Fats: 26 g
Calories: 329 Kcal

99. Strawberry, Fruity And Nutty Smoothie

Preparation Time: 5 minutes
Servings: 4 cups

Ingredients

- Strawberries: 6
- Peanuts: 1 cup
- Orange: 1
- Pineapple: 1 cup chopped
- Water: 1 cup

Directions:

1. Add all the ingredients to the blender
2. Blend to form a smooth consistency

Nutrition:
Carbs: 18.2 g
Protein: 8 g
Fats: 18.2 g
Calories: 258 Kcal

100. Sunflower Seed Butter Smoothie

Preparation Time: 5 minutes
Servings: 2

Ingredients

- Coconut milk: 1 cup
- Frozen banana: 1 small sliced
- Sunflower Seed butter: 2 tbsp
- Spinach: 1/2 cup sliced

Directions:
1. Add all the ingredients to the blender
2. Blend to form a smooth consistency

Nutritional Facts

Carbs: 33.1 g
Protein: 13.2 g
Fats: 18.0 g
Calories: 335 Kcal

101. Tropical Paradise Smoothie

Preparation Time: 5 minutes
Servings: 2

Ingredients

- Frozen peeled banana: 1 thinly sliced
- Fresh mango: ½ cup diced
- Ice cubes: 4
- Full-fat coconut milk: 1 cup
- Pineapple chunks: ¾ cup
- Ground ginger: 1/8 tsp
- Chia seeds: 1 tbsp
- Toasted shredded coconut: 2 tbsp for topping

Directions:
1. Add all the ingredients to the blender except toasted coconuts
2. Blend to make smooth
3. Top with toasted coconuts and serve

Nutritional Facts

Carbs: 33.3 g

Protein: 8 g
Fats: 26.4 g
Calories: 359 Kcal

102. Veggie Omelet

Preparation time: 15 minutes
Cooking time: 23 minutes
Servings: 2
Ingredients:

- 8 ounces fresh asparagus, trimmed and cut into 1-inch pieces
- ¼ of red bell pepper, seeded
- ¼ of green bell pepper, seeded
- 1 tablespoon fresh chives, chopped
- ¾ cup water
- ½ cup superfine chickpea flour
- 1 tablespoon chia seeds
- 2 tablespoons nutritional yeast
- ½ teaspoon baking powder
- 1 teaspoon dried basil, crushed
- ¼ teaspoon ground turmeric
- ¼ teaspoon red pepper flakes, crushed
- Salt and ground black pepper, as required
- 1 small tomato, chopped

Directions:
1. In a pan of the lightly salted boiling water, add the asparagus and Cooking Time: for about 5-7 minutes or until crisp tender.
2. Drain the asparagus well and set aside.
3. Meanwhile, in a bowl, add the bell peppers, chives and water and mix.
4. In another bowl, add the remaining ingredients except tomato and mix well.
5. Add the water mixture into the bowl of flour mixture and mix until well combined.
6. Set aside for at least 10 minutes.

7. Lightly, grease a large nonstick skillet and heat over medium heat
8. Add ½ of the mixture and with the back of a spoon, smooth it.
9. Sprinkle half of the tomato over mixture evenly.
10. Cover the skillet tightly and Cooking Time: for about 4 minutes.
11. Now, place half of cooked asparagus over one side of omelet.
12. Carefully, fold the other half over asparagus to cover it.
13. Cover the skillet and Cooking Time: for 3-4 minutes more.
14. Repeat with the remaining mixture.
15. Serve warm.

Tip:
1. In a resealable plastic bag, place the cooled omelet slices and seal the bag.
2. Refrigerate for about 2-3 days.
3. Reheat in the microwave on High for about 1 minute before serving.

Nutrition:
Calories: 271, Fats: 5.2g, Carbs: 44.7g, Fiber: 15.8g, Sugar: 9.5g, Proteins: 18.2g, Sodium: 104mg

103. Veggies Quiche

Preparation time: 15 minutes
Cooking time: 1 hour; Servings: 4
Ingredients:

- 1 cup water
- Pinch of salt
- 1/3 cup bulgur wheat
- ¾ tablespoon light sesame oil
- 1½ cups fresh cremini mushrooms, sliced
- 2 cups fresh broccoli, chopped
- 1 yellow onion, chopped
- 16 ounces firm tofu, pressed and cubed
- ¾ tablespoon white miso
- 1¼ tablespoons tahini
- 1 tablespoon soy sauce

Directions:
1. Preheat the oven to 350 degrees F. Grease a pie dish.
2. In a pan, add the water over medium heat and salt bring to a boil.
3. Stir in the bulgur and again bring to a boil.
4. Reduce the heat to low and simmer, covered for about 12-15 minutes or until all the liquid is absorbed.
5. Remove from the heat and let it cool slightly.
6. Now, place the cooked bulgur into the pie dish evenly and with your fingers, press into the bottom.
7. Bake for about 12 minutes.
8. Remove from the oven and let it cool slightly.
9. Meanwhile, in a skillet, heat oil over medium heat.
10. Add the mushrooms, broccoli and onion and Cooking Time: for about 10 minutes, stirring occasionally.
11. Remove from the heat and transfer into a large bowl to cool slightly.
12. Meanwhile, in a food processor, add the remaining ingredients and pulse until smooth.
13. Transfer the tofu mixture into the bowl with veggie mixture and mix until well combined.
14. Place the veggie mixture over the baked crust evenly.
15. Bake for about 30 minutes or until top becomes golden brown.
16. Remove from the oven and set aside for at least 10 minutes.
17. With a sharp knife, cut into 4 equal sized slices and serve.

1. In a reseal able plastic bag, place the cooled quiche slices and seal the bag.
2. Refrigerate for about 2-4 days.
3. Reheat in the microwave on High for about 1 minute before serving.

Nutrition:

Calories: 212, Fats: 10.4g, Carbs: 19.6g, Fiber: 5.7g, Sugar: 3.4g, Proteins: 14.4g, Sodium: 425mg

104. Simple Bread

Preparation time: 15 minutes
Cooking time: 40 minutes
Servings: 16
Ingredients:

- 2 teaspoons maple syrup
- 2 cups warm water
- 4 cups whole-wheat flour
- 1 tablespoon instant yeast
- ½ teaspoon salt

Directions:

1. In a cup, dissolve the maple syrup in warm water.
2. In a large bowl, add the flour, yeast and salt and mix well.
3. Add the maple syrup mixture and mix until a sticky dough forms.
4. Transfer the dough into a greased 9×5-inch loaf pan.
5. Cover the loaf pan and set aside for about 20 minutes.
6. Preheat the oven to 390 degrees F.
7. Uncover the loaf pan and bake for about 40 minutes or until a toothpick inserted in the center comes out clean.
8. Remove the pan from oven and place onto a wire rack to cool for about 20 minutes.
9. Carefully, remove the bread from the loaf pan and place onto the wire rack to cool completely before slicing.

10. With a sharp knife, cut the bread loaf into desired sized slices and serve.
11. Meal Preparation time: Tip:
12. In a resealable plastic bag, place the bread and seal the bag after squeezing out the excess air.
13. Keep the bread away from direct sunlight and preserve in a cool and dry place for about 1-2 days.

Nutrition:

Calories: 118, Fats: 0.3g, Carbs: 24.7g, Fiber: 1g, Sugar: 0.6g, Proteins: 3.5g, Sodium: 76mg

105. Quinoa Bread

Preparation time: 15 minutes
Cooking time: 1½ hours
Servings: 12
Ingredients:

- 1¾ cups uncooked quinoa, soaked overnight and rinsed
- ¼ cup chia seeds, soaked in ½ cup of water overnight
- ½ teaspoon bicarbonate soda
- Salt, as required
- ¼ cup olive oil
- ½ cup water
- 1 tablespoon fresh lemon juice

Directions:

1. Preheat the oven to 320 degrees F. Line a loaf pan with parchment paper.
2. In a food processor, add all the ingredients and pulse for about 3 minutes.
3. Place the mixture into the prepared loaf pan evenly.
4. Bake for about 1½ hours or until a toothpick inserted in the center comes out clean.
5. Remove the pan from oven and place onto a wire rack to cool for about 20 minutes.
6. Carefully, remove the bread from the

loaf pan and place onto the wire rack to cool completely before slicing.

7. With a sharp knife, cut the bread loaf into desired sized slices and serve.

Meal Preparation time: Tip:

8. In a resealable plastic bag, place the bread and seal the bag after squeezing out the excess air.

9. Keep the bread away from direct sunlight and preserve in a cool and dry place for about 1-2 days.

Nutrition:

Calories: 137, Fats: 6.5g, Carbs: 16.9g, Fiber: 2.6g, Sugar: 0g, Proteins: 4g, Sodium: 20mg

106. Fruity Oatmeal Muffins

Preparation time: 15 minutes
Cooking time: 20 minutes
Servings: 6
Ingredients:

- ½ cup hot water
- ¼ cup ground flaxseeds
- 1 banana, peeled and sliced
- 1 apple, peeled, cored and chopped roughly
- 2 cups rolled oats
- ½ cup walnuts, chopped
- ½ cup raisins
- ¼ teaspoon baking soda
- 2 tablespoons ground cinnamon
- ½ cup almond milk
- ¼ cup maple syrup

Directions:

1. Preheat the oven to 350 degrees F. Line a 12 cups muffin tin with paper liners.

2. In a bowl, add water and flaxseed and beat until well combined. Set aside for about 5 minutes.

3. In a blender, add the flaxseed mixture and remaining all ingredients except

blueberries and pulse till smooth and creamy.

4. Transfer the mixture into prepared muffin cups evenly.

5. Bake for about 20 minutes or until a toothpick inserted in the center comes out clean.

6. Remove the muffin tin from oven and place onto a wire rack to cool for about 10 minutes.

7. Carefully invert the muffins onto the wire rack to cool completely before serving.

Meal Preparation time: Tip:

8. Carefully invert the muffins onto a wire rack to cool completely.

9. Line 1-2 airtight containers with paper towels.

10. Arrange muffins over paper towel in a single layer.

11. Cover the muffins with another paper towel.

12. Refrigerate for about 2-3 days.

13. Reheat in the microwave on High for about 2 minutes before serving.

Nutrition:

Calories: 351, Fats: 14.4g, Carbs: 51.8g, Fiber: 8.2g, Sugar: 22.4g, Proteins: 8.2g, Sodium: 61mg

MAINS

107. Grilled tempeh with green beans

Preparation Time: 15 minutes
Serving: 4
If there is ever a dish that can replace the essence of BBQ, this would be it! Plus the extra ingredients of green beans.

Ingredients

- 1 tbsp plant butter, melted
- 1 lb tempeh, sliced into 4 pieces
- 1 lb green beans, trimmed
- Salt and black pepper to taste
- 2 sprigs thyme
- 2 tbsp olive oil
- 1 tbsp pure corn syrup
- 1 lemon, juiced

Directions

1. Preheat a grill pan over medium heat and brush with the plant butter.
2. Season the tempeh and green beans with the salt, black pepper, and place the thyme in the pan. Grill the tempeh and green beans on both sides until golden brown and tender, 10 minutes.
3. Transfer to serving plates.
4. In a small bowl, whisk the olive oil, corn syrup, lemon juice, and drizzle all over the food.
5. Serve warm.

Nutrition:
Calories 352
Fats 22.5g | Carbs 21.8g
Protein 22.6g

108. Tofu Fajita Bowl

Preparation Time: 5minutes
Cooking Time: 10minutes
Servings: 4
Ingredients:

- 2 tbsp olive oil
- 1½ lb tofu, cut into strips
- Salt and ground black pepper to taste
- 2 tbsp Tex-Mex seasoning
- 1 small iceberg lettuce, chopped
- 2 large tomatoes, deseeded and chopped
- 2 avocados, halved, pitted, and chopped
- 1 green bell pepper, deseeded and thinly sliced
- 1 yellow onion, thinly sliced
- 4 tbsp fresh cilantro leaves
- ½ cup shredded dairy- free parmesan cheese blend
- 1 cup plain unsweetened yogurt

Directions:

1. Heat the olive oil in a medium skillet over medium heat, season the tofu with salt, black pepper, and Tex-Mex seasoning. Fry in the oil on both sides until golden and cooked, 5 to 10 minutes. Transfer to a plate.
2. Divide the lettuce into 4 serving bowls, share the tofu on top, and add the tomatoes, avocados, bell pepper, onion, cilantro, and cheese.
3. Top with dollops of plain yogurt and serve immediately with low carb tortillas.

Nutrition:
Calories:263, Total Fat:26.4g, Saturated Fat:8.8g, Total Carbs:4g, Dietary Fiber:1g, Sugar:3g, Protein:4g, Sodium:826mg

109. Indian Style Tempeh Bake

Preparation Time: 10minutes
Cooking Time: 26minutes
Servings: 4
Ingredients:

- 3 tbsp unsalted butter
- 6 tempeh, cut into 1-inch cubes
- Salt and ground black pepper to taste
- 2 ½ tbsp garam masala
- 1 cup baby spinach, tightly pressed
- 1¼ cups coconut creaminutes
- 1 tbsp fresh cilantro, finely chopped

Directions:

1. Preheat the oven to 350 F and grease a baking dish with cooking spray. Set aside.
2. Heat the ghee in a medium skillet over medium heat, season the tempeh with salt and black pepper, and Cooking Time: in the oil on both sides until golden on the outside, 6 minutes.
3. Mix in half of the garam masala and transfer the tempeh (with juicesinto the baking dish.
4. Add the spinach, and spread the coconut cream on top. Bake in the oven for 20 minutes or until the cream is bubbly.
5. Remove the dish, garnish with cilantro, and serve with cauliflower couscous.

Nutrition:
Calories:598, Total Fat:56g, Saturated Fat:18.8g, Total Carbs12:g, Dietary Fiber:3g, Sugar:5g, Protein:15g, Sodium:762mg

110. Tofu- Seitan Casserole

Preparation Time: 10minutes
Cooking Time: 20minutes
Servings: 4
Ingredients:

- 1 tofu, shredded
- 7 oz seitan, chopped
- 8 oz dairy- free cream cheese (vegan
- 1 tbsp Dijon mustard
- 1 tbsp plain vinegar
- 10 oz shredded cheddar cheese
- Salt and ground black pepper to taste

Directions:

1. Preheat the oven to 350 F and grease a baking dish with cooking spray. Set aside.
2. Spread the tofu and seitan in the bottom of the dish.
3. In a small bowl, mix the cashew cream, Dijon mustard, vinegar, and two-thirds of the cheddar cheese. Spread the mixture on top of the tofu and seitan, season with salt and black pepper, and cover with the remaining cheese.
4. Bake in the oven for 15 to 20 minutes or until the cheese melts and is golden brown.
5. Remove the dish and serve with steamed collards.

Nutrition:
Calories475:, Total Fat:41.2g, Saturated Fat:12.3g, Total Carbs:6g, Dietary Fiber:3g, Sugar:2g, Protein:24g, Sodium:755mg

111. Ginger Lime Tempeh

Preparation Time: 10 minutes
Cooking Time: 40 minutes
Servings: 4
Ingredients:

- 5 kaffir lime leaves
- 1 tbsp cumin powder
- 1 tbsp ginger powder
- 1 cup plain unsweetened yogurt
- 2 lb tempeh
- Salt and ground black pepper to taste

- 1 tbsp olive oil
- 2 limes, juiced

Directions:

1. In a large bowl, combine the kaffir lime leaves, cumin, ginger, and plain yogurt. Add the tempeh, season with salt, and black pepper, and mix to coat well. Cover the bowl with a plastic wrap and marinate in the refrigerator for 2 to 3 hours.
2. Preheat the oven to 350 F and grease a baking sheet with cooking spray.
3. Take out the tempeh and arrange on the baking sheet. Drizzle with olive oil, lime juice, cover with aluminum foil, and slow-Cooking Time: in the oven for 1 to 1 ½ hours or until the tempeh cooks within.
4. Remove the aluminum foil, turn the broiler side of the oven on, and brown the top of the tempeh for 5 to 10 minutes.
5. Take out the tempeh and serve warm with red cabbage slaw.

Nutrition:
Calories:285, Total Fat:25.6g, Saturated Fat:13.6g, Total Carbs:7g, Dietary Fiber:2g, Sugar:2g, Protein:11g, Sodium:772mg

112. Tofu Mozzarella

Preparation Time: 10minutes
Cooking Time: 35minutes
Servings: 4
Ingredients:
- 1½ lb tofu, halved lengthwise
- Salt and ground black pepper to taste
- 2 eggs
- 2 tbsp Italian seasoning
- 1 pinch red chili flakes
- ½ cup sliced Pecorino Romano cheese
- ¼ cup fresh parsley, chopped

- 4 tbsp butter
- 2 garlic cloves, minced
- 2 cups crushed tomatoes
- 1 tbsp dried basil
- Salt and ground black pepper to taste
- ½ lb sliced mozzarella cheese

Directions:

1. Preheat the oven to 400 F and grease a baking dish with cooking spray. Set aside.
2. Season the tofu with salt and black pepper; set aside.
3. In a medium bowl, whisk the eggs with the Italian seasoning, and red chili flakes. In a plate, combine the Pecorino Romano cheese with parsley.
4. Melt the butter in a medium skillet over medium heat.
5. Quickly dip the tofu in the egg mixture and then dredge generously in the cheese mixture. Place in the butter and fry on both sides until the cheese melts and is golden brown, 8 to 10 minutes. Place on a plate and set aside.
6. Sauté the garlic in the same pan and mix in the tomatoes. Top with the basil, salt, and black pepper, and Cooking Time: for 5 to 10 minutes. Pour the sauce into the baking dish.
7. Lay the tofu pieces in the sauce and top with the mozzarella cheese. Bake in the oven for 10 to 15 minutes or until the cheese melts completely.
8. Remove the dish and serve with leafy green salad.

Nutrition:
Calories:140, Total Fat:13.2g, Saturated Fat:7.1g, Total Carbs:2g, Dietary Fiber:0g, Sugar:0g, Protein:3g, Sodium:78mg1

113. Seitan Meatza With Kale

Preparation Time: 10minutes
Cooking Time: 22minutes
Servings: 4
Ingredients:

- 1 lb ground seitan
- Salt and black pepper to taste
- 2 cups powdered Parmesan cheese
- ¼ tsp onion powder
- ¼ tsp garlic powder
- ½ cup unsweetened tomato sauce
- 1 tsp white vinegar
- ½ tsp liquid smoke
- ¼ cup baby kale, chopped roughly
- 1 cup mozzarella cheese

Directions:

1. Preheat the oven to 400 F and line a medium pizza pan with parchment paper and grease with cooking spray. Set aside.
2. In a medium bowl, combine the seitan, salt, black pepper, and parmesan cheese. Spread the mixture on the pizza pan to fit the shape of the pan. Bake in the oven for 15 minutes or until the meat cooks.
3. Meanwhile in a medium bowl, mix the onion powder, garlic powder, tomato sauce, vinegar, and liquid smoke. Remove the meat crust from the oven and spread the tomato mixture on top. Add the kale and sprinkle with the mozzarella cheese.
4. Bake in the oven for 7 minutes or until the cheese melts.
5. Take out from the oven, slice, and serve warm.

Nutrition:
Calories:601, Total Fat:51.8g, Saturated Fat:16.4g, Total Carbs:18g, Dietary Fiber:5g, Sugar:3g, Protein:23g, Sodium:398mg

114. Taco Tempeh Casserole

Preparation Time: 10minutes
Cooking Time: 20minutes
Servings: 4
Ingredients:

- 1 Tempeh, shredded
- 1/3 cup vegan mayonnaise
- 8 oz dairy- free cream cheese (vegan
- 1 yellow onion, sliced
- 1 yellow bell pepper, deseeded and chopped
- 2 tbsp taco seasoning
- ½ cup shredded cheddar cheese
- Salt and ground black pepper to taste

Directions:

1. Preheat the oven to 400 F and grease a baking dish with cooking spray.
2. Into the dish, put the tempeh, mayonnaise, cashew cream, onion, bell pepper, taco seasoning, and two-thirds of the cheese, salt, and black pepper. Mix the Ingredients and top with the remaining cheese.
3. Bake in the oven for 15 to 20 minutes or until the cheese melts and is golden brown.
4. Remove the dish, plate, and serve with lettuce leaves.

Nutrition:
Calories:132, Total Fat:11.5g, Saturated Fat4:4.3g, Total Carbs:7g, Dietary Fiber:4g, Sugar:2g, Protein:1g, Sodium:10mg

115. Broccoli Tempeh Alfredo

Preparation Time: 10minutes
Cooking Time: 15minutes
Servings: 4
Ingredients:

- 6 slices tempeh, chopped
- 2 tbsp butter
- 4 tofu, cut into 1-inch cubes

- Salt and ground black pepper to taste
- 4 garlic cloves, minced
- 1 cup baby kale, chopped
- 1 ½ cups full- fat heavy creaminutes
- 1 medium head broccoli, cut into florets
- ¼ cup shredded parmesan cheese

Directions:

1. Put the tempeh in a medium skillet over medium heat and fry until crispy and brown, 5 minutes. Spoon onto a plate and set aside.
2. Melt the butter in the same skillet, season the tofu with salt and black pepper, and Cooking Time: on both sides until goldern- brown. Spoon onto the tempeh's plate and set aside.
3. Add the garlic to the skillet, sauté for 1 minute.
4. Mix in the full- fat heavy cream, tofu, and tempeh, and kale, allow simmering for 5 minutes or until the sauce thickens.
5. Meanwhile, pour the broccoli into a large safe-microwave bowl, sprinkle with some water, season with salt, and black pepper, and microwave for 2 minutes or until the broccoli softens.
6. Spoon the broccoli into the sauce, top with the parmesan cheese, stir and Cooking Time: until the cheese melts. Turn the heat off.
7. Spoon the mixture into a serving platter and serve warm.

Nutrition:
Calories:193, Total Fat:20.1g, Saturated Fat:12.5g, Total Carbs:3g, Dietary Fiber:0g, Sugar:2g, Protein:1g, Sodium:100mg

116. Avocado Seitan

Preparation Time: 10 minutes
Cooking Time: 2 hours 15 minutes
Servings: 4
Ingredients:

- 1 white onion, finely chopped
- ¼ cup vegetable stock
- 3 tbsp coconut oil
- 3 tbsp tamari sauce
- 3 tbsp chili pepper
- 1 tbsp red wine vinegar
- Salt and ground black pepper to taste
- 2 lb Seitan
- 1 large avocado, halved and pitted
- ½ lemon, juiced

Directions:

1. In a large pot, combine the onion, vegetable stock, coconut oil, tamari sauce, chili pepper, red wine vinegar, salt, black pepper. Add the seitan, close the lid, and Cooking Time: over low heat for 2 hours.
2. Scoop the avocado pulp into a bowl, add the lemon juice, and using a fork, mash the avocado into a puree. Set aside.
3. When ready, turn the heat off and mix in the avocado. Adjust the taste with salt and black pepper.
4. Spoon onto a serving platter and serve warm.

Nutrition:
Calories:412, Total Fat:43g, Saturated Fat:37g, Total Carbs:9g, Dietary Fiber:3g, Sugar:0g, Protein:5g, Sodium:12mg

117. Seitan Mushroom Burgers

Preparation Time: 15 minutes
Cooking Time: 13 minutes
Servings: 4
Ingredients:

- 1 ½ lb ground seitan
- Salt and ground black pepper to taste
- 1 tbsp unsweetened tomato sauce
- 6 large Portobello caps, destemmed
- 1 tbsp olive oil
- 6 slices cheddar cheese

For topping:
- 4 lettuce leaves
- 4 large tomato slices
- ¼ cup mayonnaise

Directions:
1. In a medium bowl, combine the seitan, salt, black pepper, and tomato sauce. Using your hands, mold the mixture into 4 patties, and set aside.
2. Rinse the mushrooms under running water and pat dry.
3. Heat the olive oil in a medium skillet; place in the Portobello caps and Cooking Time: until softened, 3 to 4 minutes. Transfer to a serving plate and set aside.
4. Put the seitan patties in the skillet and fry on both sides until brown and compacted, 8 minutes. Place the vegan cheddar slices on the food, allow melting for 1 minute and lift each patty onto each mushroom cap.
5. Divide the lettuce on top, then the tomato slices, and add some mayonnaise.
6. Serve immediately.

Nutrition:
Calories:304, Total Fat:29g, Saturated Fat:23.5g, Total Carbs:8g, Dietary Fiber:3g, Sugar:1g, Protein:8g, Sodium:8mg

118. Taco Tempeh Stuffed Peppers

Preparation Time: 15 minutes
Cooking Time: 41 minutes
Servings: 6
Ingredients:
- 6 yellow bell peppers, halved and deseeded
- 1 ½ tbsp olive oil
- Salt and ground black pepper to taste
- 3 tbsp butter
- 3 garlic cloves, minced
- ½ white onion, chopped
- 2 lbs. ground tempeh
- 3 tsp taco seasoning
- 1 cup riced broccoli
- ¼ cup grated cheddar cheese
- Plain unsweetened yogurt for serving

Directions:
1. Preheat the oven to 400 F and grease a baking dish with cooking spray. Set aside.
2. Drizzle the bell peppers with the olive oil and season with some salt. Set aside.
3. Melt the butter in a large skillet and sauté the garlic and onion for 3 minutes. Stir in the tempeh, taco seasoning, salt, and black pepper. Cooking Time: until the meat is no longer pink, 8 minutes.
4. Mix in the broccoli until adequately incorporated. Turn the heat off.
5. Spoon the mixture into the peppers, top with the cheddar cheese, and place the peppers in the baking dish. Bake in the oven until the cheese melts and is bubbly, 30 minutes.
6. Remove the dish from the oven and plate the peppers. Top with the palin yogurt and serve warm.

Nutrition:
Calories:251, Total Fat:22.5g, Saturated Fat:3.8g, Total Carbs:13g, Dietary Fiber:9g, Sugar:2g, Protein:3g, Sodium:23mg

119. Tangy Tofu Meatloaf

Preparation Time: 10 minutes
Cooking Time: 40 minutes
Servings: 6
Ingredients:

- 2 ½ lb ground tofu
- Salt and ground black pepper to taste
- 3 tbsp flaxseed meal
- 2 large eggs
- 2 tbsp olive oil
- 1 lemon,1 tbsp juiced
- ¼ cup freshly chopped parsley
- ¼ cup freshly chopped oregano
- 4 garlic cloves, minced
- Lemon slices to garnish

Directions:

1. Preheat the oven to 400 F and grease a loaf pan with cooking spray. Set aside.
2. In a large bowl, combine the tofu, salt, black pepper, and flaxseed meal. Set aside.
3. In a small bowl, whisk the eggs with the olive oil, lemon juice, parsley, oregano, and garlic. Pour the mixture onto the mix and combine well.
4. Spoon the tofu mixture into the loaf pan and press to fit into the pan. Bake in the middle rack of the oven for 30 to 40 minutes.
5. Remove the pan, tilt to drain the meat's liquid, and allow cooling for 5 minutes.
6. Slice, garnish with some lemon slices and serve with braised green beans.

Nutrition:

Calories:238, Total Fat:26.3g, Saturated Fat:14.9g, Total Carbs:1g, Dietary Fiber:0g, Sugar:0g, Protein:1g, Sodium:183mg

120. Vegan Bacon Wrapped Tofu With Buttered Spinach

Preparation Time: 5 minutes
Cooking Time: 20 minutes
Servings: 4
Ingredients:
For the bacon wrapped tofu:

- 4 tofu
- 8 slices vegan bacon
- Salt and black pepper to taste
- 2 tbsp olive oil

For the buttered spinach:

- 2 tbsp butter
- 1 lb spinach
- 4 garlic cloves
- Salt and ground black pepper to taste

Directions:
For the bacon wrapped tofu:

1. Preheat the oven to 450 F.
2. Wrap each tofu with two vegan bacon slices, season with salt and black pepper, and place on the baking sheet. Drizzle with the olive oil and bake in the oven for 15 minutes or until the vegan bacon browns and the tofu cooks within.

For the buttered spinach:

1. Meanwhile, melt the butter in a large skillet, add and sauté the spinach and garlic until the leaves wilt, 5 minutes. Season with salt and black pepper.
2. Remove the tofu from the oven and serve with the buttered spinach.

Nutrition:
Calories:260, Total Fat:24.7g, Saturated Fat:14.3g, Total Carbs:4g, Dietary Fiber:0g, Sugar:2g, Protein:6g, Sodium:215mg

121. Veggie & Tofu Kebabs

Preparation Time: 15 minutes
Cooking Time: 12 minutes
Servings: 4
Ingredients:

- 2 cloves garlic, minced
- ¼ cup balsamic vinegar
- ¼ cup olive oil
- 1 tablespoon Italian seasoning
- Salt and pepper to taste
- 1 onion, sliced into quarters
- 12 medium mushrooms
- 16 cherry tomatoes
- 1 zucchini, sliced into rounds
- 1 cup tofu, cubed
- 4 cups cauliflower rice

Directions:

1. In a bowl, mix the garlic, vinegar, oil, Italian seasoning, salt and pepper.
2. Toss the vegetable slices and tofu in the mixture.
3. Marinate for 1 hour.
4. Thread into 8 skewers and grill for 12 minutes, turning once or twice.
5. Add cauliflower rice into 4 food containers.
6. Add 2 kebab skewers on top of each container of cauliflower rice.
7. Reheat kebabs in the grill before serving.

Nutritional Value:
Calories 58
Total Fat 2 g
Saturated Fat 0 g
Cholesterol 0 mg
Sodium 84 mg
Total Carbohydrate 9 g
Dietary Fiber 2 g
Total Sugars 5 g
Protein 2 g

Potassium 509 mg

122. Carrot And Radish Slaw With Sesame Dressing

Preparation Time: 10 minutes
Cooking Time: 0 minute
Servings: 4
Ingredients:

- 2 tablespoons sesame oil, toasted
- 3 tablespoons rice vinegar
- ½ teaspoon sugar
- 2 tablespoons low sodium tamari
- 1 cup carrots, sliced into strips
- 2 cups radishes, sliced
- 2 tablespoons fresh cilantro, chopped
- 2 teaspoons sesame seeds, toasted

Directions:

1. Mix the oil, vinegar, sugar and tamari in a bowl.
2. Add the carrots, radishes and cilantro.
3. Toss to coat evenly.
4. Let sit for 10 minutes.
5. Transfer to a food container.

Nutritional Value:
Calories 98
Total Fat 8 g
Saturated Fat 1 g
Cholesterol 0 mg
Sodium 336 mg
Total Carbohydrate 6 g
Dietary Fiber 2 g
Total Sugars 3 g
Protein 2 g
Potassium 241 mg

123. Spicy Snow Pea And Tofu Stir Fry

Preparation Time: 20 minutes
Cooking Time: 20 minutes
Servings: 4
Ingredients:

- 1 cup unsalted natural peanut butter
- 2 teaspoons brown sugar
- 2 tablespoons reduced-sodium soy sauce
- 2 teaspoons hot sauce
- 3 tablespoons rice vinegar
- 14 oz. tofu
- 4 teaspoons oil
- 1/4 cup onion, sliced
- 2 tablespoons ginger, grated
- 3 cloves garlic, minced
- 1/2 cup broccoli, sliced into florets
- 1/2 cup carrot, sliced into sticks
- 2 cups fresh snow peas, trimmed
- 2 tablespoons water
- 2 cups brown rice, cooked
- 4 tablespoons roasted peanuts (unsalted

Directions:
1. In a bowl, mix the peanut butter, sugar, soy sauce, hot sauce and rice vinegar.
2. Blend until smooth and set aside.
3. Drain the tofu and sliced into cubes.
4. Pat dry with paper towel.
5. Add oil to a pan over medium heat.
6. Add the tofu and Cooking Time: for 2 minutes or until brown on all sides.
7. Transfer the tofu to a plate.
8. Add the onion, ginger and garlic to the pan.
9. Cooking Time: for 2 minutes.
10. Add the broccoli and carrot.
11. Cooking Time: for 5 minutes.
12. Stir in the snow peas.
13. Pour in the water and cover.
14. Cooking Time: for 4 minutes.
15. Add the peanut sauce to the pan along with the tofu.
16. Heat through for 30 seconds.
17. In a food container, add the brown rice and top with the tofu and vegetable stir fry.
18. Top with roasted peanuts.

Nutritional Value:
Calories 514
Total Fat 27 g
Saturated Fat 4 g
Cholesterol 0 mg
Sodium 376 mg
Total Carbohydrate 49 g
Dietary Fiber 7 g
Total Sugars 12 g
Protein 22 g
Potassium 319 mg

124. Roasted Veggies In Lemon Sauce

Preparation Time: 15 minutes
Cooking Time: 20 minutes
Servings: 5
Ingredients:
- 2 cloves garlic, sliced
- 1 ½ cups broccoli florets
- 1 ½ cups cauliflower florets
- 1 tablespoon olive oil
- Salt to taste
- 1 teaspoon dried oregano, crushed
- ¾ cup zucchini, diced
- ¾ cup red bell pepper, diced
- 2 teaspoons lemon zest

Directions:
1. Preheat your oven to 425 degrees F.
2. In a baking pan, add the garlic, broccoli and cauliflower.
3. Toss in oil and season with salt and oregano.
4. Roast in the oven for 10 minutes.
5. Add the zucchini and bell pepper to the pan.
6. Stir well.

7. Roast for another 10 minutes.
8. Sprinkle lemon zest on top before serving.
9. Transfer to a food container and reheat before serving.

Nutritional Value:
Calories 52
Total Fat 3 g
Saturated Fat 0 g
Cholesterol 0 mg
Sodium 134 mg
Total Carbohydrate 5 g
Dietary Fiber 2 g
Total Sugars 2 g
Protein 2 g
Potassium 270 mg

125. Lunch Recipes

Potato Bean Quesadillas
Preparation time: 10 minutes
Cooking time: 10 minutes
Servings: 4
Ingredients:

- 4 whole-wheat tortillas
- 2 potatoes, boiled, cubed
- 200g refried beans
- 1 teaspoon chili powder
- ½ teaspoon dried oregano
- ¼ teaspoon garlic powder
- 120g spinach
- 1 onion, thinly sliced
- 2 cloves garlic, minced
- 30ml tamari sauce
- 45g nutritional yeast
- Salt and pepper, to taste

Directions:
1. Heat a splash of olive oil in a skillet.
2. Add onion and Cooking Time: over medium heat for 10 minutes, or until the onion is caramelized.
3. Add the garlic and Cooking Time: 1 minute.
4. Add spinach and toss gently.
5. Add tamari sauce and Cooking Time: 1 minutes.
6. Reheat the refried beans with nutritional yeast, chili, oregano, and garlic powder, in a microwave, on high for 1 minute.
7. Mash the potatoes and spread over tortilla.
8. Top the mashed potatoes with spinach mixture and refried beans.
9. Season to taste and place another tortilla on top.
10. Heat large skillet over medium-high heat.
11. Heat the tortilla until crispy. Flip and heat the other side.
12. Cut the tortilla in half and serve.

Nutrition:
Calories 232
Total Fat 2.1g
Total Carbohydrate 44.2g
Dietary Fiber 10.4g
Total Sugars 3g
Protein 12.4g

126. Lemon Pepper Pasta

Preparation time: 5 minutes
Cooking time: 20 minutes
Servings: 4
Ingredients:

- 300g pasta, any kind, without eggs
- 400ml unsweetened soy milk
- 100g soy cream cheese
- 45g blanched almonds
- 45g nutritional yeast
- 1 teaspoon lemon zest, finely grated
- ¼ teaspoon lemon pepper
- 30ml olive oil

- 2 clove garlic, minced
- 5 capers, rinsed, chopped
- 10g parsley, chopped

Directions:

1. Cooking Time: the pasta, according to the package directions, in a pot filled with salted boiling water.
2. Strain the pasta and reserve 230ml cooking liquid.
3. Combine soy milk, soy cheese, almonds, nutritional yeast, lemon zest, and pepper lemon in a food blender.
4. Blend until smooth. Place aside.
5. Heat olive oil in a skillet.
6. Add the garlic, and Cooking Time: until very fragrant, for 1 minute.
7. Pour in the soy milk mixture and reserved pasta cooking liquid.
8. Bring to a boil, and reduce heat.
9. Stir in chopped capers and simmer 6-8 minutes or until creamy. Remove from the heat and stir in cooked pasta.
10. Toss the pasta gently to coat with the sauce.
11. Serve pasta, garnished with chopped parsley.

Nutrition:

Calories 489

Total Fat 23g

Total Carbohydrate 53.5g

Dietary Fiber 5.9g

Total Sugars 2.4g

Protein 20.4g

127. Lentils Salad With Lemon Tahini Dressing

Preparation time: 10 minutes

Cooking time: 30 minutes

Servings: 4

Ingredients:

- 225g green lentils, picked, rinsed
- 1 clove garlic, minced
- ¼ teaspoon ground cumin
- 5ml olive oil
- 1 red onion, finely diced
- 75g dried apricots, chopped
- 1 small red bell pepper, seeded, chopped
- 1 small green bell pepper, seeded, chopped
- 1 small yellow bell pepper, seeded, chopped
- 1 small cucumber, diced
- 20g sunflower seeds
- Salt and pepper, to taste

Lemon dressing:

- 1 lemon, juiced
- 30g tahini
- 5g chopped coriander
- Salt, to taste

Directions:

1. Place rinsed lentils in a saucepan.
2. Add enough water to cover.
3. Bring to a boil and skim off any foam. Add garlic and cumin.
4. Reduce heat and simmer the lentils for 30 minutes.
5. In the meantime, make the dressing by combining all the ingredients together.
6. Heat olive oil in a skillet. Add onion and bell peppers. Cooking Time: stirring over medium-high heat for 5 minutes.
7. Remove from the heat.
8. Drain the lentils and toss in a large bowl with the cooked vegetables, apricots, cucumber, and sunflower seeds. Season to taste.
9. Drizzle with dressing and serve.

Nutrition:

Calories 318

Total Fat 7g

Total Carbohydrate 49.2g
Dietary Fiber 20.8g
Total Sugars 7.9g
Protein 18.1g

128. Spanish Chickpea Spinach Stew

Preparation time: 10 minutes
Cooking time: 25 minutes
Servings: 4
Ingredients:
- 1 splash olive oil
- 1 small onion, chopped
- 2 cloves garlic
- 5g cumin powder
- 5g smoked paprika
- ¼ teaspoon chili powder
- 235ml water
- 670g can diced tomatoes
- 165g cooked chickpeas (or can chickpeas
- 60g baby spinach
- Salt, to taste
- A handful of chopped coriander, to garnish
- 20g slivered almonds, to garnish
- 4 slices toasted whole-grain bread, to serve with

Directions:
1. Heat olive oil in a saucepan over medium-high heat.
2. Add onion and Cooking Time: until browned, for 7-8 minutes.
3. Add garlic, cumin, paprika, and chili powder.
4. Cooking Time: 1 minute.
5. Add water and scrape any browned bits.
6. Add the tomatoes and chickpeas. Season to taste and reduce heat.

7. Simmer the soup for 10 minutes.
8. Stir in spinach and Cooking Time: 2 minutes.
9. Ladle soup in a bowl. Sprinkle with cilantro and almonds.
10. Serve with toasted bread slices.

Nutrition:
Calories 369
Total Fat 9.7g
Total Carbohydrate 67.9g
Dietary Fiber 19.9g
Total Sugars 13.9g
Protein 18g

129. Lentils Bolognese With Soba Noodles

Preparation time: 10 minutes
Cooking time: 15 minutes (plus 25 for lentils
Servings: 4
Ingredients:
Bolognese:
- 100g red lentils
- 1 bay leaf
- Splash of olive oil
- 1 small onion, diced
- 1 large stalk celery, sliced
- 3 cloves garlic, minced
- 230ml tomato sauce or fresh pureed tomatoes
- 60ml red wine or vegetable stock (if you do not like wine
- 1 tablespoon fresh basil, chopped
- Salt and pepper, to taste

Soba noodles:
- 280g soba noodles

Directions:
1. Cooking Time: the lentils; place lentils and bay leaf in a saucepan.
2. Cover with water, so the water is 2-inches above the lentils.

3. Bring to a boil over medium-high heat.
4. Reduce heat and simmer the lentils for 25 minutes.
5. Drain the lentils and discard the bay leaf.
6. Heat a splash of olive oil in a saucepan.
7. Add onion, and Cooking Time: 6 minutes.
8. Add celery and Cooking Time: 2 minutes.
9. Add garlic and Cooking Time: 2 minutes.
10. Add the tomatoes and wine. Simmer the mixture for 5 minutes.
11. Stir in the lentils and simmer 2 minutes.
12. Remove the Bolognese from the heat and stir in basil.
13. In the meantime, Cooking Time: the soba noodles according to package directions.
14. Serve noodles with lentils Bolognese.

Nutrition:
Calories 353
Total Fat 0.9g
Total Carbohydrate 74g
Dietary Fiber 9g
Total Sugars 4.2g
Protein 17.7g

130. Red Burgers

Preparation time: 10 minutes
Cooking time: 50 minutes
Servings: 4
Ingredients:
Patties:

- 2 large beets, peeled, cubed
- 1 red onion, cut into chunks
- 115g red kidney beans
- 85g red cooked quinoa
- 2 cloves garlic, minced
- 30g almond meal
- 20g ground flax
- 10ml lemon juice
- ½ teaspoon ground cumin
- ½ teaspoon red pepper flakes
- Salt, to taste
- 4 whole-meal burger buns

Tahini Guacamole:

- 1 avocado, pitted, peeled
- 45ml lime juice
- 30g tahini sauce
- 5g chopped coriander

Directions:
1. Preheat oven to 190C/375F.
2. Toss beet and onion with a splash of olive oil.
3. Season with salt. Bake the beets for 30 minutes.
4. Transfer the beets and onion into a food blender.
5. Add the beans and blend until coarse. You do not want a completely smooth mixture.
6. Stir in quinoa, garlic, almond meal, flax seeds, lemon juice, cumin, and red pepper flakes.
7. Shape the mixture into four patties.
8. Transfer the patties to a baking sheet, lined with parchment paper.
9. Bake the patties 20 minutes, flipping halfway through.
10. In the meantime, make the tahini guac; mash the avocado with lime juice in a bowl.
11. Stir in tahini and coriander. Season to taste.
12. To serve; place the patty in the bun, top with guacamole and serve.

Nutrition:

Calories 343
Total Fat 16.6g
Total Carbohydrate 49.1g
Dietary Fiber 14.4g
Total Sugars 8.1g
Protein 15g

131. Hemp Falafel With Tahini Sauce

Preparation time: 10 minutes
Cooking time: 10 minutes
Servings: 6
Ingredients:

- 80g raw hemp hearts
- 4g chopped cilantro
- 4g chopped basil
- 2 cloves garlic, minced
- 2g ground cumin seeds
- 3g chili powder
- 14g flax meal + 30ml filtered water
- Sea salt and pepper, to taste
- Avocado or coconut oil, to fry

Sauce:

- 115g tahini
- 60ml fresh lime juice
- 115ml filtered water
- 30ml extra-virgin olive oil
- Sea salt, to taste
- A good pinch ground cumin seeds

Directions:
1. Mix flax with filtered water in a small bowl.
2. Place aside for 10 minutes.
3. In meantime, combine raw hemp hearts, cilantro, basil, garlic, cumin, chili, and seasonings in a food processor.
4. Process until just comes together. Add the flax seeds mixture and process until finely blended and uniform.
5. Heat approximately 2 tablespoons avocado oil in a skillet. Shape 1 tablespoon mixture into balls and fry for 3-4 minutes or until deep golden brown.
6. Remove from the skillet and place on a plate lined with paper towels.
7. Make the sauce; combine all ingredients in a food blender. Blend until smooth and creamy.
8. Serve falafel with fresh lettuce salad and tahini sauce.

Nutrition:
Calories 347
Total Fat 29.9g
Total Carbohydrate 7.2g
Dietary Fiber 4.3g
Total Sugars 0.2g
Protein 13.8g

132. Tempeh Skewers With Dressing

Preparation time: 20 minutes
Cooking time: 10 minutes
Servings: 6
Ingredients:

- 445g tempeh, cut into fingers
- 155ml unsweetened almond milk
- 100g almond flour
- 8g paprika
- 4g garlic powder
- 3g dried basil
- Salt and pepper, to taste
- 15ml olive oil

Finger sauce:

- 60ml melted coconut oil
- 80g hot sauce
- 10 drops Stevia

Dressing:

- 230g vegan mayonnaise

- 115g vegan sour cream
- 1 clove garlic, minced
- 2g chopped dill
- 2g chopped chives
- 1g onion powder
- Salt and pepper, to taste

Directions:

1. Cut the tempeh into slices/fingers. Arrange onto bamboo skewers, soaked in water 30 minutes.
2. Bring a pot of water to a boil. Add tempeh and boil 15 minutes. Drain and place aside.
3. Heat oven to 200C/400F.
4. Pour almond milk into a bowl. Combine almond flour and spices into a separate bowl.
5. Dip the tempeh into almond milk, and coat with the almond flour mixture.
6. Grease baking sheet with coconut oil. Arrange the tempeh fingers onto a baking sheet.
7. Bake the tempeh 10 minutes. In the meantime, make the sauce.
8. Melt coconut oil in a saucepan. Add hot sauce and simmer 5minutes. Add Stevia and remove from the heat.
9. Make the dressing by combining all ingredients together.
10. Toss the tempeh with hot sauce. Serve with prepared dressing.

Nutrition:
Calories 351
Total Fat 29.3g
Total Carbohydrate 9.9g
Dietary Fiber 1g
Total Sugars 0.2g
Protein 15.5g

133. White Bean Salad With Spicy Sauce

Preparation time: 15 minutes
Servings: 4
Ingredients:

- 450g can white beans, rinsed, drained or cooked beans
- 1 avocado, peeled, chopped
- 6 cherry tomatoes, quartered
- 1 red onion, thinly sliced

Sauce:

- 80g cashews, soaked in water 4 hours
- 30ml extra-virgin olive oil
- 30ml lemon juice
- 70ml water
- 10g Dijon mustard
- 5g pure maple syrup
- 1 clove garlic
- ½ teaspoon cayenne pepper
- ½ teaspoon paprika powder
- 1 pinch salt

Directions:

1. Make the sauce; rinse and drain cashews and place in a food processor.
2. Add the remaining ingredients, olive oil, lemon juice, water, mustard, garlic, cayenne, paprika, and salt.
3. Process until smooth and creamy. Place aside.
4. Make the salad; prepared vegetables as described.
5. Toss the beans with avocado, cherry tomatoes, and red onion.
6. Drizzle with prepared dressing and toss once again.
7. Serve or refrigerate before serving.

Nutrition:
Calories 366
Total Fat 24.2g

Total Carbohydrate 31.9g
Dietary Fiber 9.5g
Total Sugars 5.6g
Protein 11g

134. Stuffed Sweet Hummus Potatoes

Preparation time: 10 minutes
Cooking time: 15 minutes
Servings: 4
Ingredients:

- 4 large sweet potatoes
- 10ml olive oil
- 200g kale, stems removed, chopped
- 300g can black beans, drained, rinsed
- 240g hummus
- 60ml water
- 5g garlic powder
- Salt and pepper, to taste
- Sour cream:
- 100g raw cashews, soaked in water for 4 hours
- 80ml water
- 15ml raw cider vinegar
- 15ml lemon juice
- 1 pinch salt

Directions:

1. Prick sweet potato with a fork or toothpick all over the surface.
2. Wrap the potato in a damp paper towel and place in a microwave.
3. Microwave the sweet potato 10 minutes or until fork tender.
4. In the meantime, heat olive oil in a skillet.
5. Add kale and Cooking Time: with a pinch of salt until wilted.
6. Add black beans and Cooking Time: 2 minutes.
7. Make the sour cream; combine all sour cream ingredients in a food processor.
8. Process until creamy. Chill briefly before serving.
9. Make a slit in each sweet potato.
10. Combine hummus, water, and garlic powder in a bowl.
11. Stuff potato with the kale-bean mixture. Top the sweet potato with hummus and a dollop of sour cream.
12. Serve.

Nutrition:
Calories 540
Total Fat 20.3g2
Total Carbohydrate 78.1g
Dietary Fiber 14.9g
Total Sugars 3g
Protein 16.6g

135. Crusted Tofu Steaks With Caramelized Onion

Preparation time: 15 minutes
Cooking time: 45 minutes
Servings: 4
Ingredients:

- 450g tofu, cut into 8 steaks/slices
- 100g graham crackers
- 80g raw cashews
- 230ml unsweetened soy milk
- 120g whole-wheat flour
- 10g garlic powder
- 10g onion powder
- 10g chili powder
- 5g lemon pepper
- 15ml olive oil
- Salt, to taste

Onion:

- 15ml grapeseed oil
- 1 large onion
- 15ml balsamic vinegar

- 15ml lemon juice
- 15ml water
- 15g maple sugar

Directions:
1. Make the tofu; preheat oven to 200C/400F and line a baking sheet with parchment paper.
2. Combine graham crackers and cashews in a food processor.
3. Process unto coarse crumbs form.
4. Transfer to a large bowl.
5. In a separate bowl, combine flour, garlic and onion powder, chili, and lemon pepper.
6. Pour the soy milk into a third bowl.
7. Coat tofu with flour, dip into milk and finally coat with the graham cracker crumbs.
8. Arrange the tofu steaks onto a baking sheet.
9. Bake the tofu for 15-20 minutes or until golden brown.
10. In the meantime, make the onion; heat grapeseed oil in a skillet.
11. Add onion and Cooking Time: over medium-high heat for 8 minutes.
12. Add balsamic, lemon juice, and maple sugar. Cooking Time: 2 minutes.
13. Add water and reduce heat. Simmer 15 minutes.
14. Serve tofu steaks with caramelized onions.

Nutrition:
Calories 617
Total Fat 29.5g
Total Carbohydrate 70.6g
Dietary Fiber 5.8g
Total Sugars 17g
Protein 23.6g

136. Spicy Beans And Rice

Preparation time: 10 minutes
Cooking time: 1 hour 10 minutes
Servings: 6
Ingredients:
- 450g dry red kidney beans, soaked overnight
- 15ml olive oil
- 1 onion, diced
- 1 red bell pepper, seeded, diced
- 1 large stalk celery, sliced
- 4 cloves garlic, minced
- 15ml hot sauce
- 5g paprika
- 2g dried thyme
- 2 g parsley, chopped
- 2 bay leaves
- 900ml vegetable stock
- 280g brown rice
- Salt and pepper, to taste

Directions:
1. Drain the beans and place aside.
2. Heat olive oil in a saucepot.
3. Add onion and bell pepper. Cooking Time: 6 minutes.
4. Add celery and Cooking Time: 3 minutes.
5. Add garlic, hot sauce, paprika, and thyme. Cooking Time: 1 minute.
6. Add the drained beans, bay leaves, and vegetable stock.
7. Bring to a boil, and reduce heat.
8. Simmer the beans for 1 hour 15 minutes or until tender.
9. In the meantime, place rice in a small saucepot. Cover the rice with 4cm water.
10. Season to taste and Cooking Time: the rice until tender, for 25 minutes.
11. To serve; transfer ¼ of the beans into

a food processor. Process until smooth.

12. Combine the processed beans with the remaining beans and ladle into a bowl.

13. Add rice and sprinkle with parsley before serving.

Nutrition:
Calories 469
Total Fat 6g
Total Carbohydrate 87.5g
Dietary Fiber 14.2g
Total Sugars 4.9g
Protein 21.1g

137. Chili Quinoa Stuffed Peppers

Preparation time: 15 minutes
Cooking time: 1 hour 5 minutes
Servings: 4
Ingredients:

- 160g quinoa
- 460ml vegetable stock
- 2 red bell peppers, cut in half, seeds and membrane removed
- 2 yellow bell peppers, cut in half, seeds, and membrane removed
- 120g salsa
- 15g nutritional yeast
- 10g chili powder
- 5g cumin powder
- 425g can black beans, rinsed, drained
- 160g fresh corn kernels
- Salt and pepper, to taste
- 1 small avocado, sliced
- 15g chopped cilantro

Directions:

1. Preheat oven to 190C/375F.
2. Brush the baking sheet with some cooking oil.
3. Combine quinoa and vegetable stock in a saucepan. Bring to a boil.
4. Reduce heat and simmer 20 minutes.
5. Transfer the quinoa to a large bowl.
6. Stir in salsa, nutritional yeast, chili powder, cumin powder, black beans, and corn. Season to taste with salt and pepper.
7. Stuff the bell pepper halves with prepared mixture.
8. Transfer the peppers onto a baking sheet, cover with aluminum foil, and bake for 30 minutes.
9. Increase heat to 200C/400F and bake the peppers for an additional 15 minutes.
10. Serve warm, topped with avocado slices, and chopped cilantro.

Nutrition:
Calories 456
Total Fat 15.4g
Total Carbohydrate 71.1g
Dietary Fiber 15.8g
Total Sugars 8.2g
Protein 17.4g

138. Spinach With Walnuts & Avocado

Preparation Time: 5 minutes
Cooking Time: 0 minute
Servings: 1
Ingredients:

- 3 cups baby spinach
- ½ cup strawberries, sliced
- 1 tablespoon white onion, chopped
- 2 tablespoons vinaigrette
- ¼ medium avocado, diced
- 2 tablespoons walnut, toasted

Directions:

1. Put the spinach, strawberries and onion in a glass jar with lid.

2. Drizzle dressing on top.
3. Top with avocado and walnuts.
4. Seal the lid and refrigerate until ready to serve.

Nutritional Value:
Calories 296
Total Fat 18 g
Saturated Fat 2 g
Cholesterol 0 mg
Sodium 195 mg
Total Carbohydrate 27 g
Dietary Fiber 10 g
Total Sugars 11 g
Protein 8 g
Potassium 103 mg

139. Vegan Tacos

Preparation Time: 20 minutes
Cooking Time: 10 minutes
Servings: 4
Ingredients:

- ½ teaspoon onion powder
- ½ teaspoon garlic powder
- 1 teaspoon chili powder
- 2 tablespoons tamari
- 16 oz. tofu, drained and crumbled
- 1 tablespoon olive oil
- 1 ripe avocado
- 1 tablespoon vegan mayonnaise
- 1 teaspoon lime juice
- Salt to taste
- 8 corn tortillas, warmed
- ½ cup fresh salsa
- 2 cups iceberg lettuce, shredded
- Pickled radishes

Directions:

1. Combine the onion powder, garlic powder, chili powder and tamari in a bowl.
2. Marinate the tofu in the mixture for

10 minutes.
3. Pour the oil in a pan over medium heat.
4. Cooking Time: the tofu mixture for 10 minutes.
5. In another bowl, mash the avocado and mix with mayo, lime juice and salt.
6. Stuff each corn tortilla with tofu mixture, mashed avocado, salsa and lettuce.
7. Serve with pickled radishes.

Nutritional Value:
Calories 360
Total Fat 21 g
Saturated Fat 3 g
Cholesterol 0 mg
Sodium 610 mg
Total Carbohydrate 33 g
Dietary Fiber 8 g
Total Sugars 4 g
Protein 17 g
Potassium 553 mg

140. Grilled Broccoli with Chili Garlic Oil

Preparation Time: 15 minutes
Cooking Time: 16 minutes
Servings: 4
Ingredients:

- 3 tablespoons olive oil, divided
- 2 tablespoons vegetable broth (unsalted
- 2 cloves garlic, sliced thinly
- 1 chili pepper, julienned
- 1 1/2 lb. broccoli, sliced into florets
- Salt and pepper to taste
- 2 lemons, sliced in half

Directions:

1. Preheat your grill to medium-high.
2. In a bowl, mix 1 tablespoon oil, garlic, broth and chili.

3. Heat in a pan over medium heat for 30 seconds.
4. In another bowl, toss the broccoli florets in salt, pepper and remaining oil.
5. Grill the broccoli florets for 10 minutes.
6. Grill the lemon slices for 5 minutes.
7. Toss the grilled broccoli and lemon in chili garlic oil.
8. Store in a food container and reheat before serving.

Nutritional Value:
Calories 164
Total Fat 11 g
Saturated Fat 1 g
Cholesterol 0 mg
Sodium 208 mg
Total Carbohydrate 12 g
Dietary Fiber 2 g
Total Sugars 4 g
Protein 6 g
Potassium 519 mg

141. Tomato Basil Pasta

Preparation Time: 5 minutes
Cooking Time: 10 minutes
Servings: 4
Ingredients:
- 2 cups low-sodium vegetable broth
- 2 cups water
- 8 oz. pasta
- 1 ½ teaspoons Italian seasoning
- 15 oz. canned diced tomatoes
- 2 tablespoons olive oil
- ½ teaspoon garlic powder
- ½ teaspoon onion powder
- ¼ teaspoon crushed red pepper
- ½ teaspoon salt
- 6 cups baby spinach

- ½ cup basil, chopped

Directions:
1. Add all the ingredients except spinach and basil in a pot over high heat.
2. Mix well.
3. Cover the pot and bring to a boil.
4. Reduce the heat.
5. Simmer for 5 minutes.
6. Add the spinach and Cooking Time: for 5 more minutes.
7. Stir in basil.
8. Transfer to a food container.
9. Microwave before serving.

Nutritional Value:
Calories 339
Total Fat 10 g
Saturated Fat 1 g
Cholesterol 0 mg
Sodium 465 mg
Total Carbohydrate 55 g
Dietary Fiber 8 g
Total Sugars 6 g
Protein 11 g
Potassium 308 mg

142. Risotto With Tomato & Herbs

Preparation Time: 10 minutes
Cooking Time: 20 minutes
Servings: 32
Ingredients:
- 2 oz. Arborio rice
- 1 teaspoon dried garlic, minced
- 3 tablespoons dried onion, minced
- 1 tablespoon dried Italian seasoning, crushed
- ¾ cup snipped dried tomatoes
- 1 ½ cups reduced-sodium chicken broth

Directions:
1. Make the dry risotto mix by

combining all the ingredients except broth in a large bowl.
2. Divide the mixture into eight resealable plastic bags. Seal the bag.
3. Store at room temperature for up to 3 months.
4. When ready to serve, pour the broth in a pot.
5. Add the contents of 1 plastic bag of dry risotto mix.
6. Bring to a boil and then reduce heat.
7. Cover the pot and simmer for 20 minutes.
8. Serve with vegetables.

Nutritional Value:
Calories 80
Total Fat 0 g
Saturated Fat 0 g
Cholesterol 0 mg
Sodium 276 mg
Total Carbohydrate 17 g
Dietary Fiber 2 g
Total Sugars 0 g
Protein 3 g
Potassium 320 mg

143. Tofu Shawarma Rice

Preparation Time: 15 minutes
Cooking Time: 15 minutes
Servings: 4
Ingredients:
- 4 cups cooked brown rice
- 4 cups cooked tofu, sliced into small cubes
- 4 cups cucumber, cubed
- 4 cups tomatoes, cubed
- 4 cups white onion, cubed
- 2 cups cabbage, shredded
- 1/2 cup vegan mayo
- 1/8 cup garlic, minced
- Garlic salt to taste

- Hot sauce

Directions:
1. Add brown rice into 4 food containers.
2. Arrange tofu, cucumber, tomatoes, white onion and cabbage on top.
3. In a bowl, mix the mayo, garlic, and garlic salt.
4. Drizzle top with garlic sauce and hot sauce before serving.

Nutritional Value:
Calories 667
Total Fat 12.6g
Saturated Fat 2.2g
Cholesterol 0mg
Sodium 95mg
Total Carbohydrate 116.5g
Dietary Fiber 9.9g
Total Sugars 9.4g
Protein 26.1g
Potassium 1138mg

144. Pesto Pasta

Preparation Time: 10 minutes
Cooking Time: 8 minutes
Servings: 2
Ingredients:
- 1 cup fresh basil leaves
- 4 cloves garlic
- 2 tablespoons walnut
- 2 tablespoons olive oil
- 1 tablespoon vegan Parmesan cheese
- 2 cups cooked penne pasta
- 2 tablespoons black olives, sliced

Directions:
1. Put the basil leaves, garlic, walnut, olive oil and Parmesan cheese in a food processor.
2. Pulse until smooth.
3. Divide pasta into 2 food containers.
4. Spread the basil sauce on top.

5. Top with black olives.
6. Store until ready to serve.

Nutritional Value:
Calories 374
Total Fat 21.1g
Saturated Fat 2.6g
Cholesterol 47mg
Sodium 92mg
Total Carbohydrate 38.6g
Dietary Fiber 1.1g
Total Sugars 0.2g
Protein 10g
Potassium 215mg

145. "Cheesy" Spinach Rolls

Preparation Time: 20 minutes
Cooking Time: 15 minutes
Servings: 6
Ingredients:

- 18 spinach leaves
- 18 vegan spring roll wrappers
- 6 slices cheese, cut into 18 smaller strips
- Water
- 1 cup vegetable oil
- 6 cups cauliflower rice
- 3 cups tomato, cubed
- 3 cups cucumber, cubed
- 1 tablespoon olive oil
- 1 teaspoon balsamic vinegar

Directions:
1. Place one spinach leaf on top of each wrapper.
2. Add a small strip of vegan cheese on top of each spinach leaf.
3. Roll the wrapper and seal the edges with water.
4. In a pan over medium high heat, add the vegetable oil.
5. Cooking Time: the rolls until golden brown.
6. Drain in paper towels.
7. Divide cauliflower rice into 6 food containers.
8. Add 3 cheesy spinach rolls in each food container.
9. Toss cucumber and tomato in olive oil and vinegar.
10. Place the cucumber tomato relish beside the rolls.
11. Seal and reheat in the microwave when ready to serve.

Nutritional Value:
Calories 746
Total Fat 38.5g
Saturated Fat 10.1g
Cholesterol 33mg
Sodium 557mg
Total Carbohydrate 86.2g
Dietary Fiber 3.8g
Total Sugars 2.6g
Protein 18g
Potassium 364mg

146. Grilled Summer Veggies

Preparation Time: 15 minutes
Cooking Time: 6 minutes
Servings: 6
Ingredients:

- 2 teaspoons cider vinegar
- 1 tablespoon olive oil
- ¼ teaspoon fresh thyme, chopped
- 1 teaspoon fresh parsley, chopped
- ¼ teaspoon fresh rosemary, chopped
- Salt and pepper to taste
- 1 onion, sliced into wedges
- 2 red bell peppers, sliced
- 3 tomatoes, sliced in half
- 6 large mushrooms, stems removed
- 1 eggplant, sliced crosswise

- 3 tablespoons olive oil
- 1 tablespoon cider vinegar

Directions:

1. Make the dressing by mixing the vinegar, oil, thyme, parsley, rosemary, salt and pepper.
2. In a bowl, mix the onion, red bell pepper, tomatoes, mushrooms and eggplant.
3. Toss in remaining olive oil and cider vinegar.
4. Grill over medium heat for 3 minutes.
5. Turn the vegetables and grill for another 3 minutes.
6. Arrange grilled vegetables in a food container.
7. Drizzle with the herbed mixture when ready to serve.

Nutritional Value:

Calories 127

Total Fat 9 g

Saturated Fat 1 g

Cholesterol 0 mg

Sodium 55 mg

Total Carbohydrate 11 g

Dietary Fiber 5 g

Total Sugars 5 g

Protein 3 g

Potassium 464 mg

147. Superfood Buddha Bowl

Preparation Time: 10 minutes

Cooking Time: 10 minutes

Servings: 4

Ingredients:

- 8 oz. microwavable quinoa
- 2 tablespoons lemon juice
- ½ cup hummus
- Water
- 5 oz. baby kale
- 8 oz. cooked baby beets, sliced
- 1 cup frozen shelled edamame (thawed
- ¼ cup sunflower seeds, toasted
- 1 avocado, sliced
- 1 cup pecans
- 2 tablespoons flaxseeds

Directions:

1. Cooking Time: quinoa according to directions in the packaging.
2. Set aside and let cool.
3. In a bowl, mix the lemon juice and hummus.
4. Add water to achieve desired consistency.
5. Divide mixture into 4 condiment containers.
6. Cover containers with lids and put in the refrigerator.
7. Divide the baby kale into 4 food containers with lids.
8. Top with quinoa, beets, edamame and sunflower seeds.
9. Store in the refrigerator until ready to serve.
10. Before serving add avocado slices and hummus dressing.

Nutritional Value:

Calories 381

Total Fat 19 g

Saturated Fat 2 g

Cholesterol 0 mg

Sodium 188 mg

Total Carbohydrate 43 g

Dietary Fiber 13 g

Total Sugars 8 g

Protein 16 g

Potassium 1,066 mg

148. Burrito & Cauliflower Rice Bowl

Preparation Time: 15 minutes
Cooking Time: 10 minutes
Servings: 4
Ingredients:

- 1 cup cooked tofu cubes
- 12 oz. frozen cauliflower rice
- 4 teaspoons olive oil
- 1 teaspoon unsalted taco seasoning
- 1 cup red cabbage, sliced thinly
- ½ cup salsa
- ¼ cup fresh cilantro, chopped
- 1 cup avocado, diced

Directions:

1. Prepare cauliflower rice according to directions in the package.
2. Toss cauliflower rice in olive oil and taco seasoning.
3. Divide among 4 food containers with lid.
4. Top with tofu, cabbage, salsa and cilantro.
5. Seal the container and chill in the refrigerator until ready to serve.
6. Before serving, add avocado slices.

Nutritional Value:
Calories 298
Total Fat 20 g
Saturated Fat 3 g
Cholesterol 0 mg
Sodium 680 mg
Total Carbohydrate 15 g
Dietary Fiber 6 g
Total Sugars 5 g
Protein 15 g
Potassium 241 mg

149. Seitan Zoodle Bowl

Preparation Time: 15 minutes
Cooking Time: 13 minutes
Servings: 4
Ingredients:

- 5 garlic cloves, minced, divided
- ¼ tsp pureed onion
- Salt and ground black pepper to taste
- 2 ½ lb Seitan, cut into strips
- 2 tbsp avocado oil
- 3 large eggs, lightly beaten
- ¼ cup vegetable broth
- 2 tbsp coconut aminos
- 1 tbsp white vinegar
- ½ cup freshly chopped scallions
- 1 tsp red chili flakes
- 4 medium zucchinis, spiralized
- ½ cup toasted pine nuts, for topping

Directions:

1. In a medium bowl, combine the half of the pureed garlic, onion, salt, and black pepper. Add the seitan and mix well.
2. Heat the avocado oil in a large, deep skillet over medium heat and add the seitan. Cooking Time: for 8 minutes. Transfer to a plate.
3. Pour the eggs into the pan and scramble for 1 minute. Spoon the eggs to the side of the seitan and set aside.
4. Reduce the heat to low and in a medium bowl, mix the vegetable broth, coconut aminos, vinegar, scallions, remaining garlic, and red chili flakes. Mix well and simmer for 3 minutes.
5. Stir in the seitan, zucchini, and eggs. Cooking Time: for 1 minute and turn the heat off. Adjust the taste with salt and black pepper.

6. Spoon the zucchini food into serving plates, top with the pine nuts and serve warm.

Nutrition:
Calories:687, Total Fat:54.5g, Saturated Fat:27.4g, Total Carbs:9g, Dietary Fiber:2g, Sugar:4g, Protein:38g, Sodium:883mg

150. Tofu Parsnip Bake

Preparation Time: 5 minutes
Cooking Time: 44 minutes
Servings: 4
Ingredients:

- 6 vegan bacon slices, chopped
- 2 tbsp butter
- ½ lb parsnips, peeled and diced
- 2 tbsp olive oil
- 1 lb ground tofu
- Salt and ground black pepper to taste
- 2 tbsp butter
- 1 cup full- fat heavy creaminutes
- 2 oz dairy- free cream cheese (vegan), softened
- 1 ¼ cups grated cheddar cheese
- ¼ cup chopped scallions

Directions:
1. Preheat the oven to 300 F and lightly grease a baking dish with cooking spray. Set aside.
2. Put the vegan bacon in a medium pot and fry on both sides until brown and crispy, 7 minutes. Spoon onto a plate and set aside.
3. Melt the butter in a large skillet and sauté the parsnips until softened and lightly browned. Transfer to the baking sheet and set aside.
4. Heat the olive oil in the same pan and Cooking Time: the tofu (seasoned with salt and black pepper). Spoon onto a plate and set aside too.

5. Add the butter, full- fat heavy cream, cashew cream, two-thirds of the cheddar cheese, salt, and black pepper to the pot. Melt the Ingredients over medium heat with frequent stirring, 7 minutes.
6. Spread the parsnips in the baking dish, top with the tofu, pour the full- fat heavy cream mixture over, and scatter the top with the vegan bacon and scallions.
7. Sprinkle the remaining cheese on top, and bake in the oven until the cheese melts and is golden, 30 minutes.
8. Remove the dish, spoon the food into serving plates, and serve immediately.

Nutrition:
Calories:534, Total Fat:56g, Saturated Fat:34.6g, Total Carbs:4g, Dietary Fiber:1g, Sugar:1g, Protein:7g, Sodium:430mg

151. Squash Tempeh Lasagna

Preparation Time: 15 minutes
Cooking Time: 40 minutes
Servings: 4
Ingredients:

- 2 tbsp butter
- 1 ½ lb ground tempeh
- Salt and ground black pepper to taste
- 1 tsp garlic powder
- 1 tsp onion powder
- 2 tbsp coconut flour
- 1 ½ cup grated mozzarella cheese
- 1/3 cup parmesan cheese
- 2 cups crumbled cottage cheese
- 1 large egg, beaten into a bowl
- 2 cups unsweetened marinara sauce
- 1 tbsp dried Italian mixed herbs
- ¼ tsp red chili flakes
- 4 large yellow squash, sliced
- ¼ cup fresh basil leaves

Directions:
1. Preheat the oven to 375 F and grease a baking dish with cooking spray. Set aside.
2. Melt the butter in a large skillet over medium heat and Cooking Time: the tempeh until brown, 10 minutes. Set aside to cool.
3. In a medium bowl, mix the garlic powder, onion powder, coconut flour, salt, black pepper, mozzarella cheese, half of the parmesan cheese, cottage cheese, and egg. Set aside.
4. In another bowl, combine the marinara sauce, mixed herbs, and red chili flakes. Set aside.
5. Make a single layer of the squash slices in the baking dish; spread a quarter of the egg mixture on top, a layer of the tempeh, then a quarter of the marinara sauce. Repeat the layering process in the same ingredient proportions and sprinkle the top with the remaining parmesan cheese.
6. Bake in the oven until golden brown on top, 30 minutes.
7. Remove the dish from the oven, allow cooling for 5 minutes, garnish with the basil leaves, slice and serve.

Nutrition:
Calories:194, Total Fat:17.4g, Saturated Fat:2.1g, Total Carbs:7g, Dietary Fiber:3g, Sugar:2g, Protein:7g, Sodium:72mg

152. Bok Choy Tofu Skillet

Preparation Time: 10 minutes
Cooking Time: 18 minutes
Servings: 4
Ingredients:
- 2 lb tofu, cut into 1-inch cubes
- Salt and ground black pepper to taste
- 4 vegan bacon slices, chopped
- 1 tbsp coconut oil
- 1 orange bell pepper, deseeded, cut into chunks
- 2 cups baby bok choy
- 2 tbsp freshly chopped oregano
- 2 garlic cloves, pressed

Directions:
1. Season the tofu with salt and black pepper, and set aside.
2. Heat a large skillet over medium heat and fry the vegan bacon until brown and crispy. Transfer to a plate.
3. Melt the coconut oil in the skillet and Cooking Time: the tofu until golden-brown and cooked through, 10 minutes. Remove onto the vegan bacon plate and set aside.
4. Add the bell pepper and bok choy to the skillet and sauté until softened, 5 minutes. Stir in the vegan bacon, tofu, oregano, and garlic. Season with salt and black pepper and Cooking Time: for 3 minutes or until the flavors incorporate. Turn the heat off.
5. Plate the dish and serve with cauliflower rice.

Nutrition:
Calories:273, Total Fat:18.7g, Saturated Fat:7.9g, Total Carbs:15g, Dietary Fiber:4g, Sugar:8g, Protein:15g, Sodium:341mg

153. Quorn Sausage Frittata

Preparation Time: 10 minutes
Cooking Time: 33 minutes
Servings: 4
Ingredients:
- 12 whole eggs
- 1 cup plain unsweetened yogurt
- Salt and ground black pepper to taste
- 1 tbsp butter
- 1 celery stalk, chopped
- 12 oz quorn sausages

- ¼ cup shredded cheddar cheese

Directions:

1. Preheat the oven to 350 F.
2. In a medium bowl, whisk the eggs, plain yogurt, salt, and black pepper.
3. Melt the butter in a large (safe ovenskillet over medium heat. Sauté the celery until soft, 5 minutes. Transfer the celery into a plate and set aside.
4. Add the quorn sausages to the skillet and Cooking Time: until brown with frequent stirring to break the lumps that form, 8 minutes.
5. Flatten the quorn sausage in the bottom of the skillet using the spoon, scatter the celery on top, pour the egg mixture all over, and sprinkle with the cheddar cheese.
6. Put the skillet in the oven and bake until the eggs set and cheese melts, 20 minutes.
7. Remove the skillet, slice the frittata, and serve warm with kale salad.

Nutrition:
Calories:293, Total Fat:27.9g, Saturated Fat:2.9g, Total Carbs:11g, Dietary Fiber:4g, Sugar:2g, Protein:5g, Sodium:20mg

154. Jamaican Jerk Tempeh

Preparation Time: 15 minutes
Cooking Time: 45 minutes
Servings: 4
Ingredients:

- ½ cup plain unsweetened yogurt
- 2 tbsp melted butter
- 2 tbsp Jamaican jerk seasoning
- Salt and black pepper to taste
- 2 lb tempeh
- 3 tbsp tofu
- ¼ cup almond meal

Directions:

1. Preheat the oven to 350 F and grease a baking sheet with cooking spray.
2. In a large bowl, combine the plain yogurt, butter, Jamaican jerk seasoning, salt, and black pepper. Add the tempeh and toss to coat evenly. Allow marinating for 15 minutes.
3. In a food processor, blend the tofu with the almond meal until finely combined. Pour the mixture onto a wide plate.
4. Remove the tempeh from the marinade, shake off any excess liquid, and coat generously in the tofu mixture. Place on the baking sheet and grease lightly with cooking spray.
5. Bake in the oven for 40 to 45 minutes or until golden brown and crispy, turning once.
6. Remove the tempeh and serve warm with red cabbage slaw and parsnip fries.

Nutrition:
Calories:684, Total Fat:68g, Saturated Fat:12.1g, Total Carbs:13g, Dietary Fiber:4g, Sugar:1g, Protein:13g, Sodium:653mg

155. Zucchini Seitan Stacks

Preparation Time: 15 minutes
Cooking Time: 18 minutes
Servings: 4
Ingredients:

- 1 ½ lb seitan
- 3 tbsp almond flour
- Salt and black pepper to taste
- 2 large zucchinis, cut into 2-inch slices
- 4 tbsp olive oil
- 2 tsp Italian mixed herb blend
- ½ cup vegetable broth

Directions:

1. Preheat the oven to 400 F.
2. Cut the seitan into strips and set

aside.

3. In a zipper bag, add the almond flour, salt, and black pepper. Mix and add the seitan slices. Seal the bag and shake to coat the seitan with the seasoning.

4. Grease a baking sheet with cooking spray and arrange the zucchinis on the baking sheet. Season with salt and black pepper, and drizzle with 2 tablespoons of olive oil.

5. Using tongs, remove the seitan from the almond flour mixture, shake off the excess flour, and put two to three seitan strips on each zucchini.

6. Season with the herb blend and drizzle again with olive oil.

7. Cooking Time: in the oven for 8 minutes; remove the sheet and carefully pour in the vegetable broth. Bake further for 5 to 10 minutes or until the seitan cooks through.

8. Remove from the oven and serve warm with low carb bread.

Nutrition:
Calories:582, Total Fat:49.7g, Saturated Fat:18.4g, Total Carbs:8g, Dietary Fiber:3g, Sugar:2g, Protein:31g, Sodium:385mg

156. Curried Tofu Meatballs

Preparation Time: 5 minutes
Cooking Time: 25 minutes
Servings: 4
Ingredients:

- 3 lb ground tofu
- 1 medium yellow onion, finely chopped
- 2 green bell peppers, deseeded and chopped
- 3 garlic cloves, minced
- 2 tbsp melted butter
- 1 tsp dried parsley

- 2 tbsp hot sauce
- Salt and ground black pepper to taste
- 1 tbsp red curry powder
- 3 tbsp olive oil

Directions:

1. Preheat the oven to 400 F and grease a baking sheet with cooking spray.

2. In a bowl, combine the tofu, onion, bell peppers, garlic, butter, parsley, hot sauce, salt, black pepper, and curry powder. With your hands, form 1-inch tofu ball from the mixture and place on the greased baking sheet.

3. Drizzle the olive oil over the meat and bake in the oven until the tofu ball brown on the outside and Cooking Time: within, 20 to 25 minutes.

4. Remove the dish from the oven and plate the tofu ball.

5. Garnish with some scallions and serve warm on a bed of spinach salad with herbed vegan paneer cheese dressing.

Nutrition:
Calories:506, Total Fat:45.6g, Saturated Fat:18.9g, Total Carbs:11g, Dietary Fiber:1g, Sugar:1g, Protein:19g, Sodium:794mg

157. Spicy Mushroom Collard Wraps

Preparation Time: 10 minutes
Cooking Time: 16 minutes
Servings: 4
Ingredients:

- 2 tbsp avocado oil
- 1 large yellow onion, chopped
- 2 garlic cloves, minced
- Salt and ground black pepper to taste
- 1 small jalapeño pepper, deseeded and finely chopped
- 1 ½ lb mushrooms, cut into 1-inch cubes

- 1 cup cauliflower rice
- 2 tsp hot sauce
- 8 collard leaves
- ¼ cup plain unsweetened yogurt for topping

Directions:
1. Heat 2 tablespoons of avocado oil in a large deep skillet; add and sauté the onion until softened, 3 minutes.
2. Pour in the garlic, salt, black pepper, and jalapeño pepper; Cooking Time: until fragrant, 1 minute.
3. Mix in the mushrooms and Cooking Time: both sides, 10 minutes.
4. Add the cauliflower rice, and hot sauce. Sauté until the cauliflower slightly softens, 2 to 3 minutes. Adjust the taste with salt and black pepper.
5. Lay out the collards on a clean flat surface and spoon the curried mixture onto the middle part of the leaves, about 3 tablespoons per leaf. Spoon the plain yogurt on top, wrap the leaves, and serve immediately.

Nutrition:
Calories:380, Total Fat:34.8g, Saturated Fat:19.9g, Total Carbs:10g, Dietary Fiber:5g, Sugar:5g, Protein:10g, Sodium:395mg

158. Pesto Tofu Zoodles

Preparation Time: 5minutes
Cooking Time: 12minutes
Servings size 4
Ingredients:
- 2 tbsp olive oil
- 1 medium white onion, chopped
- 1 garlic clove, minced
- 2 (14 ozblocks firm tofu, pressed and cubed
- 1 medium red bell pepper, deseeded and sliced

- 6 medium zucchinis, spiralized
- Salt and black pepper to taste
- ¼ cup basil pesto, olive oil based
- 2/3 cup grated parmesan cheese
- ½ cup shredded mozzarella cheese
- Toasted pine nuts to garnish

Directions:
1. Heat the olive oil in a medium pot over medium heat; sauté the onion and garlic until softened and fragrant, 3 minutes.
2. Add the tofu and Cooking Time: until golden on all sides then pour in the bell pepper and Cooking Time: until softened, 4 minutes.
3. Mix in the zucchinis, pour the pesto on top, and season with salt and black pepper. Cooking Time: for 3 to 4 minutes or until the zucchinis soften a little bit. Turn the heat off and carefully stir in the parmesan cheese.
4. Dish into four plates, share the mozzarella cheese on top, garnish with the pine nuts, and serve warm.

Nutrition:
Calories:79, Total Fat:6.2g, Saturated Fat:3.7g, Total Carbs:5g, Dietary Fiber:2g, Sugar:3g, Protein:2g, Sodium:54mg

159. Cheesy Mushroom Pie

Preparation Time: 12minutes
Cooking Time: 43minutes
Servings: 4
Ingredients:

For the piecrust:
- ¼ cup almond flour + extra for dusting
- 3 tbsp coconut flour
- ½ tsp salt
- ¼ cup butter, cold and crumbled
- 3 tbsp erythritol

- 1 ½ tsp vanilla extract
- 4 whole eggs

For the filling:
- 2 tbsp butter
- 1 medium yellow onion
- 2 garlic cloves, minced
- 2 cups mixed mushrooms, chopped
- 1 green bell pepper, deseeded and diced
- 1 cup green beans, cut into 3 pieces each
- Salt and black pepper to taste
- ¼ cup coconut creaminutes
- 1/3 cup vegan sour creaminutes
- ½ cup almond milk
- 2 eggs, lightly beaten
- ¼ tsp nutmeg powder
- 1 tbsp chopped parsley
- 1 cup grated parmesan cheese

Directions:

For the pastry crust:
1. Preheat the oven to 350 F and grease a pie pan with cooking spray
2. In a large bowl, mix the almond flour, coconut flour, and salt.
3. Add the butter and mix with an electric hand mixer until crumbly. Add the erythritol and vanilla extract until mixed in. Then, pour in the eggs one after another while mixing until formed into a ball.
4. Flatten the dough a clean flat surface, cover in plastic wrap, and refrigerate for 1 hour.
5. After, lightly dust a clean flat surface with almond flour, unwrap the dough, and roll out the dough into a large rectangle, ½ - inch thickness and fit into a pie pan.
6. Pour some baking beans onto the

pastry and bake in the oven until golden. Remove after, pour the beans, and allow cooling.

For the filling:
1. Meanwhile, melt the butter in a skillet and sauté the onion and garlic until softened and fragrant, 3 minutes. Add the mushrooms, bell pepper, green beans, salt and black pepper; Cooking Time: for 5 minutes.
2. In a medium bowl, beat the coconut cream, vegan sour cream, milk, and eggs. Season with black pepper, salt, and nutmeg. Stir in the parsley and cheese.
3. Spread the mushroom mixture in the baked pastry and spread the cheese filling on top. Place the pie in the oven and bake for 30 to 35 minutes or until a toothpick inserted into the pie comes out clean and golden on top.
4. Remove, let cool for 10 minutes, slice, and serve with roasted tomato salad.

Nutrition:
Calories:120, Total Fat:9.2g, Saturated Fat:2.3g, Total Carbs:7g, Dietary Fiber:3g, Sugar:3g, Protein:5g, Sodium:17mg

160. Tofu Scallopini With Lemon

Preparation Time: 5minutes
Cooking Time: 21minutes
Servings: 4
Ingredients:
- 1½ lb thin cut tofu chops, boneless
- Salt and ground black pepper to taste
- 1 tbsp avocado oil
- 3 tbsp butter
- 2 tbsp capers
- 1 cup vegetable broth
- ½ lemon, juiced + 1 lemon, sliced
- 2 tbsp freshly chopped parsley

Directions:

1. Heat the avocado oil in a large skillet over medium heat. Season the tofu chops with salt and black pepper; Cooking Time: in the oil on both sides until brown and cooked through, 12 to 15 minutes. Transfer to a plate, cover with another plate, and keep warm.
2. Add the butter to the pan to melt and Cooking Time: the capers until hot and sizzling stirring frequently to avoid burning, 3 minutes.
3. Pour in the vegetable broth and lemon juice, use a spatula to scrape any bits stuck to the bottom of the pan, and allow boiling until the sauce reduces by half.
4. Add the tofu back to the sauce, arrange the lemon slices on top, and sprinkle with half of the parsley. Allow simmering for 3 minutes.
5. Plate the food, garnish with the remaining parsley, and serve warm with creamy mashed cauliflower.

Nutrition:
Calories:214, Total Fat:15.6g, Saturated Fat:2.5g, Total Carbs:12g, Dietary Fiber:2g, Sugar:6g, Protein:9g, Sodium:280mg

161. Tofu Chops With Green Beans And Avocado Sauté

Preparation Time: 10minutes
Cooking Time: 22 minutes
Servings: 4
Ingredients:

For the tofu chops:
- 2 tbsp avocado oil
- 4 slices firm tofu
- Salt and ground black pepper to taste

For the green beans and avocado sauté:
- 2 tbsp avocado oil

- 1 ½ cups green beans
- 2 large avocados, halved, pitted, and chopped
- Salt and ground black pepper to taste
- 6 green onions, chopped
- 1 tbsp freshly chopped parsley

Directions:

For the tofu chops:
Heat the avocado oil in a medium skillet, season the tofu with salt and black pepper, and fry in the oil on both sides until brown, and cooked through, 12 to 15 minutes. Transfer to a plate and set aside in a warmer for serving.

For the green beans and avocado sauté:
1. Heat the avocado oil in a medium skillet, add and sauté the green beans until sweating and slightly softened, 10 minutes. Mix in the avocados (don't worry if they mash up a bit), season with salt and black pepper, and the half of the green onions. Warm the avocados for 2 minutes. Turn the heat off.
2. Dish the sauté into serving plates, garnish with the remaining green onions and parsley, and serve with the tofu chops.

Nutrition:
Calories:503, Total Fat:41.9g, Saturated Fat:14.5g, Total Carbs:18g, Dietary Fiber:2g, Sugar:4g, Protein:19g, Sodium:314mg

162. Mexican Quinoa And Lima Bean Bowls

Preparation Time: 30 minutes
Serving: 4
A bowl filled with Mexican flavors with lima beans and quinoa for the perfect combo! Full of flavors and spices.

Ingredients
- 1 tbsp olive oil

- 1 lb extra firm tofu, pressed and cut into 1-inch cubes
- Salt and black pepper to taste
- 1 medium yellow onion, finely diced
- ½ cup cauliflower florets
- 1 jalapeño pepper, minced
- 2 garlic cloves, minced
- 1 tbsp red chili powder
- 1 tsp cumin powder
- 1 (8 ozcan sweet corn kernels, drained
- 1 (8 ozcan lima beans, rinsed and drained
- 1 cup quick-cooking quinoa
- 1 (14 ozcan diced tomatoes
- 2 ½ cups vegetable broth
- 1 cup grated homemade plant-based cheddar cheese
- 2 tbsp chopped fresh cilantro
- 2 limes, cut into wedges for garnishing
- 1 medium avocado, pitted, sliced and peeled

Directions

1. Heat olive oil in a pot and Cooking Time: the tofu until golden brown, 5 minutes. Season with salt, pepper, and mix in onion, cauliflower, and jalapeño pepper. Cooking Time: until the vegetables soften, 3 minutes. Stir in garlic, chili powder, and cumin powder; Cooking Time: for 1 minute.
2. Mix in sweet corn kernels, lima beans, quinoa, tomatoes, and vegetable broth. Simmer until the quinoa absorbs all the liquid, 10 minutes. Fluff quinoa. Top with the plant-based cheddar cheese, cilantro, lime wedges, and avocado. Serve warm.

Nutrition:
Calories 414
Fats 20.3g| Carbs 45.9g

Protein 20.8g

163. Creole Tempeh Rice Bowls

Preparation Time: 50 minutes
Serving: 4
Tempeh with vegetable over rice makes it delicious and healthy.

Ingredients

- 2 tbsp olive oil
- 1 ½ cups crumbled tempeh
- 1 tsp Creole seasoning
- 2 red bell peppers, deseeded and sliced
- 1 cup brown rice
- 2 cups vegetable broth
- Salt to taste
- 1 lemon, zested and juiced
- 1 (8 ozcan black beans, drained and rinsed
- 2 chives, chopped
- 2 tbsp freshly chopped parsley

Directions

1. Heat the olive oil in a medium pot and Cooking Time: in the tempeh until golden brown, 5 minutes.
2. Season with the Creole seasoning and stir in the bell peppers. Cooking Time: until the peppers slightly soften, 3 minutes.
3. Stir in the brown rice, vegetable broth, salt, and lemon zest.
4. Cover and Cooking Time: until the rice is tender and all the liquid is absorbed, 15 to 25 minutes.
5. Mix in the lemon juice, beans, and chives. Allow warming for 3 to 5 minutes and dish the food.
6. Garnish with the parsley and serve warm.

Nutrition:
Calories 216
Fats 13.9g| Carbs 13.8g

Protein 12.7g

164. Seitan Pesto Panini

Preparation Time: 15 minutes + 30 minutes refrigeration
Serving: 4
This is a delicious panini made from all plant sources.

Ingredients

For the seitan:

- 2/3 cup basil pesto
- ½ lemon, juiced
- 1 garlic clove, minced
- 1/8 tsp salt
- 1 cup chopped seitan

For the panini:

- 3 tbsp basil pesto
- 8 thick slices whole-wheat ciabatta
- Olive oil for brushing
- 8 slices plant-based mozzarella cheese
- 1 small yellow bell pepper, deseeded and chopped
- ¼ cup grated Parmesan cheese

Directions

For the seitan:

1. In a medium bowl, mix the pesto, lemon juice, garlic, and salt. Add the seitan and coat well with the marinade. Cover with a plastic wrap and marinate in the refrigerator for 30 minutes.
2. Preheat a large skillet over medium heat and remove the seitan from the fridge. Cooking Time: the seitan in the skillet until brown and cooked through, 2 to 3 minutes. Turn the heat off.

To make the panini:

1. Preheat a panini press to medium heat. In a small bowl, mix the pesto in the inner parts of two slices of bread. On the outer parts, apply some olive oil and place a slice with (the olive oil side downin the press.
2. Lay 2 slices of plant-based mozzarella cheese on the bread, spoon some seitan on top. Sprinkle with some bell pepper, and some plant-based Parmesan cheese. Cover with another bread slice.
3. Close the press and grill the bread for 1 to 2 minutes. Flip the bread, and grill further for 1 minute or until the cheese melts and golden brown on both sides. Serve warm.

Nutrition:
Calories 608
Fats 44.1g| Carbs 17g
Protein 37.6g

165. Creamy Fettucine With Peas

Preparation Time: 25 minutes
Serving: 4
This one is a dish made to taste fantastic. The tip for success is covering or coating the noodles in so much lushness.

Ingredients

- 16 oz whole-wheat fettuccine
- Salt and black pepper to taste
- ¾ cup flax milk
- ½ cup cashew butter, room temperature
- 1 tbsp olive oil
- 2 garlic cloves, minced
- 1 ½ cups frozen peas
- ½ cup chopped fresh basil

Directions

1. Add the fettuccine and 10 cups of water to a large pot, and Cooking Time: over medium heat until al

dente, 10 minutes. Drain the pasta through a colander and set aside. In a bowl, whisk the flax milk, cashew butter, and salt until smooth. Set aside.

2. Heat the olive oil in a large skillet and sauté the garlic until fragrant, 30 seconds. Mix in the peas, fettuccine, and basil. Toss well until the pasta is well-coated in the sauce and season with some black pepper. Dish the food and serve warm.

Nutrition:

Calories 654

Fats 23.7g| Carbs 101.9g

Protein 18.2g

166. Buckwheat Cabbage Rolls

Preparation Time: 30 minutes

Serving: 4

Ingredients

- 2 tbsp plant butter
- 2 cups extra firm tofu, pressed and crumbled
- ½ medium sweet onion, finely chopped
- 2 garlic cloves, minced
- Salt and black pepper to taste
- 1 cup buckwheat groats
- 1 ¾ cups vegetable stock
- 1 bay leaf
- 2 tbsp chopped fresh cilantro + more for garnishing
- 1 head Savoy cabbage, leaves separated (scraps kept)
- 1 (23 ozcanned chopped tomatoes

Directions

1. Melt the plant butter in a large bowl and Cooking Time: the tofu until golden brown, 8 minutes. Stir in the onion and garlic until softened and

fragrant, 3 minutes. Season with salt, black pepper and mix in the buckwheat, bay leaf, and vegetable stock.

2. Close the lid, allow boiling, and then simmer until all the liquid is absorbed. Open the lid; remove the bay leaf, adjust the taste with salt, black pepper, and mix in the cilantro.

3. Lay the cabbage leaves on a flat surface and add 3 to 4 tablespoons of the cooked buckwheat onto each leaf. Roll the leaves to firmly secure the filling.

4. Pour the tomatoes with juices into a medium pot, season with a little salt, black pepper, and lay the cabbage rolls in the sauce. Cooking Time: over medium heat until the cabbage softens, 5 to 8 minutes. Turn the heat off and dish the food onto serving plates. Garnish with more cilantro and serve warm.

Nutrition:

Calories 1147

Fats 112.9g| Carbs 25.6g

Protein 23.8g

167. Bbq Black Bean Burgers

Preparation Time: 20 minutes

Serving: 4

Say hello to your new winning burger.

Ingredients

- 3 (15 ozcans black beans, drained and rinsed
- 2 tbsp whole-wheat flour
- 2 tbsp quick-cooking oats
- ¼ cup chopped fresh basil
- 2 tbsp pure barbecue sauce
- 1 garlic clove, minced
- Salt and black pepper to taste
- 4 whole-grain hamburger buns, split

For topping:
- Red onion slices
- Tomato slices
- Fresh basil leaves
- Additional barbecue sauce

Directions
1. In a medium bowl, mash the black beans and mix in the flour, oats, basil, barbecue sauce, garlic salt, and black pepper until well combined. Mold 4 patties out of the mixture and set aside.
2. Heat a grill pan to medium heat and lightly grease with cooking spray.
3. Cooking Time: the bean patties on both sides until light brown and cooked through, 10 minutes.
4. Place the patties between the burger buns and top with the onions, tomatoes, basil, and some barbecue sauce.
5. Serve warm.

Nutrition:
Calories 589
Fats 17.7g| Carbs 80.9g
Protein 27.9g

168. Nutty Tofu Loaf

Preparation Time: 65 minutes
Serving: 4

Ingredients
- 2 tbsp olive oil + extra for brushing
- 2 white onions, finely chopped
- 4 garlic cloves, minced
- 1 lb firm tofu, pressed and crumbled
- 2 tbsp soy sauce
- ¾ cup chopped mixed nuts
- ¼ cup flaxseed meal
- 1 tbsp sesame seeds
- 1 cup chopped mixed bell peppers

- Salt and black pepper to taste
- 1 tbsp Italian seasoning
- ½ tsp pure date syrup
- ½ cup tomato sauce

Directions
1. Preheat the oven to 350 F and grease an 8 x 4-inch loaf pan with olive oil.
2. Heat 1 tbsp of olive oil in a small skillet and sauté the onion and garlic until softened and fragrant, 2 minutes.
3. Pour the onion mixture into a large bowl and mix with the tofu, soy sauce, nuts, flaxseed meal, sesame seeds, bell peppers, salt, black pepper, Italian seasoning, and date syrup until well combined.
4. Spoon the mixture into the loaf pan, press to fit and spread the tomato sauce on top.
5. Bake the tofu loaf in the oven for 45 minutes to 1 hour or until well compacted.
6. Remove the loaf pan from the oven, invert the tofu loaf onto a chopping board, and cool for 5 minutes. Slice and serve warm.

Nutrition:
Calories 544
Fats 39.2g| Carbs 30.4g
Protein 25g

169. Taco Rice Bowls

Preparation Time: 50 minutes
Serving: 4

Ingredients
- 2 tbsp olive oil
- 2 cups chopped soy chorizo
- 1 tsp taco seasoning
- 2 green bell peppers, deseeded and sliced
- 1 cup brown rice

- 2 cups vegetable broth
- Salt to taste
- ¼ cup salsa
- 1 lemon, zested and juiced
- 1 (8 ozcan pinto beans, drained and rinsed
- 1 (7 ozcan sweet corn kernels, drained
- 2 green onions, chopped
- 2 tbsp freshly chopped parsley

Directions

1. Heat the olive oil in a medium pot and Cooking Time: the soy chorizo until golden brown, 5 minutes.
2. Season with the taco seasoning and stir in the bell peppers; Cooking Time: until the peppers slightly soften, 3 minutes.
3. Stir in the brown rice, vegetable broth, salt, salsa, and lemon zest.
4. Close the lid and Cooking Time: the food until the rice is tender and all the liquid is absorbed, 15 to 25 minutes.
5. Mix in the lemon juice, pinto beans, corn kernels, and green onions. Allow warming for 3 to 5 minutes and dish the food.
6. Garnish with the parsley and serve warm.

Nutrition:
Calories 253
Fats 8.4g
Carbs 32.7g
Protein 15.5g

170. Red Sauce Mushroom Pizza

Preparation Time: 40 minutes
Serving: 4

Ingredients

For the crust:
- 2 tbsp flax seed powder + 6 tbsp water
- ½ cup tofu mayonnaise
- ¾ cup whole-wheat flour
- 1 tsp baking powder
- ½ tsp salt

For the topping:
- 1 cup sliced mixed mushrooms
- 2 tbsp olive oil
- 1 tbsp basil pesto
- Salt and black pepper
- ½ cup red pizza sauce
- ¾ cup shredded plant-based Parmesan cheese

Directions

1. Preheat the oven to 350 F.
2. In a medium bowl, mix the flax seed powder with water and allow thickening for 5 minutes to make the flax egg. Mix in the tofu mayonnaise, whole-wheat flour, baking powder, and salt until dough forms. Spread the dough on a pizza pan and bake in the oven for 10 minutes or until the dough sets.
3. In a medium bowl, mix the mushrooms, olive oil, basil pesto, salt, and black pepper.
4. Remove the pizza crust spread the pizza sauce on top. Scatter mushroom mixture on the crust and top with plant-based Parmesan cheese. Bake further until the cheese melts and the mushrooms soften, 10 to 15 minutes. Remove the pizza, slice and serve.

Nutrition:
Calories 515
Fats 35g| Carbs 35.9g
Protein 16.2g

171. Sweet Quinoa Veggie Burger

Preparation Time: 35 minutes
Serving: 4

Ingredients

- 1 cup quick-cooking quinoa
- 1 tbsp olive oil
- 1 shallot, chopped
- 2 tbsp chopped fresh celery
- 1 garlic clove, minced
- 1 (15 ozcan pinto beans, drained and rinsed
- 2 tbsp whole-wheat flour
- ¼ cup chopped fresh basil
- 2 tbsp pure maple syrup
- Salt and black pepper to taste
- 4 whole-grain hamburger buns, split
- 4 small lettuce leaves for topping
- ½ cup tofu mayonnaise for topping

Directions

1. Cooking Time: the quinoa with 2 cups of water in a medium pot until liquid absorbs, 10 to 15 minutes.
2. Meanwhile, heat the olive oil in a medium skillet over medium heat and sauté the shallot, celery, and garlic until softened and fragrant, 3 minutes.
3. Transfer the quinoa and shallot mixture to a medium bowl and add the pinto beans, flour, basil, maple syrup, salt, and black pepper. Mash and mold 4 patties out of the mixture and set aside.
4. Heat a grill pan to medium heat and lightly grease with cooking spray. Cooking Time: the patties on both sides until light brown, compacted, and cooked through, 10 minutes. Place the patties between the burger buns and top with the lettuce and tofu mayonnaise. Serve warm.

Nutrition:
Calories 290
Fats 6.2g
Carbs 50.2g
Protein 12g

172. Green Bean And Mushroom Biryani

Preparation Time: 50 minutes
Serving: 4

Ingredients

- 1 cup brown rice
- 2 cups water
- Salt to taste
- 3 tbsp plant butter
- 3 medium white onions, chopped
- 6 garlic cloves, minced
- 1 tsp ginger puree
- 1 tbsp turmeric powder + more for dusting
- ¼ tsp cinnamon powder
- 2 tsp garam masala
- ½ tsp cardamom powder
- ½ tsp cayenne powder
- ½ tsp cumin powder
- 1 tsp smoked paprika
- 3 large tomatoes, diced
- 2 green chilies, deseeded and minced
- 1 tbsp tomato puree
- 1 cup chopped cremini mushrooms
- 1 cup chopped mustard greens
- 1 cup plant-based yogurt for topping

Directions

1. Melt the butter in a large pot and sauté the onions until softened, 3 minutes. Mix in the garlic, ginger, turmeric, cardamom powder, garam masala, cardamom powder, cayenne pepper,

cumin powder, paprika, and salt. Stir-fry while cooking until the fragrant, 1 to 2 minutes.

2. Stir in the tomatoes, green chili, tomato puree, and mushrooms. Once boiling, mix in the rice and cover with water. Cover the pot and Cooking Time: over medium heat until the liquid absorbs and the rice is tender, 15-20 minutes.

3. Open the lid and fluff in the mustard greens and half of the parsley. Dish the food, top with the coconut yogurt, garnish with the remaining parsley, and serve warm.

Nutrition:
Calories 255
Fats 16.8g | Carbs 25.6g
Protein 5.8g

173. Cabbage & Bell Pepper Skillet

Preparation Time: 30 minutes
Serving: 4
Have a good benefit from my grandmum's kitchen.

Ingredients

- 1 can (28 ozwhole plum tomatoes, undrained
- 1 lb crumbled tempeh
- 1 large yellow onion, chopped
- 1 can (8 oztomato sauce
- 2 tbsp plain vinegar
- 1 tbsp pure date sugar
- 1 tsp dried mixed herbs
- 3 large tomatoes, chopped
- ½ tsp black pepper
- 1 small head cabbage, thinly sliced
- 1 medium green bell pepper, deseeded and cut into thin strips

Directions

1. Drain the tomatoes and reserve its liquid. Chop the tomatoes and set aside.

2. Add the tempeh to a large skillet and Cooking Time: until brown, 10 minutes. Mix in the onion, tomato sauce, vinegar, date sugar, mixed herbs, and chopped tomatoes. Close the lid and Cooking Time: until the liquid reduces and the tomato softens, 10 minutes.

3. Stir in the cabbage and bell pepper; Cooking Time: until softened, 5 minutes.

4. Dish the food and serve with cooked brown rice.

Nutrition:
Calories 403
Fats 16.9g
Carbs 44.1g
Protein 27.3g

174. Mixed Bean Burgers With Cashew Cheese

Preparation Time: 30 minutes
Serving: 4

Ingredients

- 1 (15 ozcan chickpea, drained and rinsed
- 1 (15 ozcan pinto beans, drained and rinsed
- 1 (15 ozcan red kidney beans, drained and rinsed
- 2 tbsp whole-wheat flour
- ¼ cup dried mixed herbs
- ¼ tsp hot sauce
- ½ tsp garlic powder
- Salt and black pepper to taste
- 4 slices cashew cheese
- 4 whole-grain hamburger buns, split
- 4 small lettuce leaves for topping

Directions

1. In a medium bowl, mash the chickpea, pinto beans, kidney beans and mix in the flour, mixed herbs, hot sauce, garlic powder, salt, and black pepper. Mold 4 patties out of the mixture and set aside.
2. Heat a grill pan to medium heat and lightly grease with cooking spray.
3. Cooking Time: the bean patties on both sides until light brown and cooked through, 10 minutes.
4. Lay a cashew cheese slice on each and allow slight melting, 2 minutes.
5. Remove the patties between the burger buns and top with the lettuce and serve warm.

Nutrition:
Calories 456
Fats 16.8g
Carbs 56.1g
Protein 24g

175. Beans, Tomato & Corn Quesadillas

Preparation Time: 35 minutes
Serving: 4

Ingredients

- 1 tsp olive oil
- 1 small onion, chopped
- ½ medium red bell pepper, deseeded and chopped
- 1 (7 ozcan chopped tomatoes
- 1 (7 ozcan black beans, drained and rinsed
- 1 (7 ozcan sweet corn kernels, drained
- 4 whole-wheat tortillas
- 1 cup grated plant-based cheddar cheese

Directions

1. Heat the olive oil in a medium skillet and sauté the onion and bell pepper until softened, 3 minutes.
2. Mix in the tomatoes, black beans, sweet corn, and Cooking Time: until the tomatoes soften, 10 minutes. Season with salt and black pepper.
3. Heat another medium skillet over medium heat and lay in one tortilla. Spread a quarter of the tomato mixture on top, scatter a quarter of the plant cheese on the sauce, and cover with another tortilla. Cooking Time: until the cheese melts. Flip and Cooking Time: further for 2 minutes.
4. Transfer to a plate and make one more piece using the remaining ingredients.
5. Cut each tortilla set into quarters and serve immediately.

Nutrition:
Calories 197
Fats 6.4g
Carbs 30.2g
Protein 6.6g

176. Bean & Rice Burritos

Preparation Time: 50 minutes
Serving: 4

Ingredients

- 1 cups brown rice
- Salt and black pepper to taste
- 1 tbsp olive oil
- 1 medium red onion, chopped
- 1 medium green bell pepper, deseeded and diced
- 2 garlic cloves, minced
- 1 tbsp chili powder
- 1 tsp cumin powder
- 1/8 tsp red chili flakes
- 1 (15 ozcan black beans, rinsed and drained

- 4 (8-inchwhole-wheat flour tortillas, warmed
- 1 cup salsa
- 1 cup coconut cream for topping
- 1 cup grated plant-based cheddar cheese for topping

Directions

1. Add 2 cups of water and brown rice to medium pot, season with some salt, and Cooking Time: over medium heat until the water absorbs and the rice is tender, 15 to 20 minutes.
2. Heat the olive oil in a medium skillet over medium heat and sauté the onion, bell pepper, and garlic until the softened and fragrant, 3 minutes.
3. Mix in the chili powder, cumin powder, red chili flakes, and season with salt and black pepper. Cooking Time: for 1 minute or until the food releases fragrance. Stir in the brown rice, black beans, and allow warming through, 3 minutes.
4. Lay the tortillas on a clean, flat surface and divide the rice mixture in the center of each. Top with the salsa, coconut cream, and plant cheddar cheese. Fold the sides and ends of the tortillas over the filling to secure. Serve immediately.

Nutrition:
Calories 421
Fats 29.1g
Carbs 37g
Protein 9.3g

177. Baked Sweet Potatoes With Corn Salad

Preparation Time: 35 minutes
Serving: 4

Ingredients

For the baked sweet potatoes:

- 3 tbsp olive oil
- 4 medium sweet potatoes, peeled and cut into ½-inch cubes
- 2 limes, juiced
- Salt and black pepper to taste
- ¼ tsp cayenne pepper
- 2 scallions, thinly sliced

For the corn salad:

- 1 (15 ozcan sweet corn kernels, drained
- ½ tbsp, plant butter, melted
- 1 large green chili, deseeded and minced
- 1 tsp cumin powder

Directions

For the baked sweet potatoes:

1. Preheat the oven to 400 F and lightly grease a baking sheet with cooking spray.
2. In a medium bowl, add the sweet potatoes, lime juice, salt, black pepper, and cayenne pepper. Toss well and spread the mixture on the baking sheet. Bake in the oven until the potatoes soften, 20 to 25 minutes.
3. Remove from the oven, transfer to a serving plate, and garnish with the scallions.

For the corn salad:

In a medium bowl, mix the corn kernels, butter, green chili, and cumin powder. Serve the sweet potatoes with the corn salad.

Nutrition:
Calories 372
Fats 20.7g
Carbs 41.7g
Protein 8.9g

178. Cheesy Broccoli Casserole

Preparation Time: 50 minutes
Serving: 4

You can make this broccoli during the holidays or any occasion. It's fabulous and super delicious.

Ingredients

- 1 tbsp olive oil
- 2 cups broccoli florets
- 1 (10 ozcan cream of mushroom soup
- 1 cup tofu mayonnaise
- Salt and black pepper to taste
- 3 tbsp coconut cream
- 1 medium red onion, chopped
- 2 cups grated plant-based cheddar cheese
- ¾ cup whole-wheat bread crumbs
- 3 tbsp plant butter, melted

Directions

1. Preheat the oven to 350 F.
2. Heat the olive oil in a medium skillet and sauté the broccoli florets until softened, 8 minutes.
3. Turn the heat off and mix in the mushroom soup, mayonnaise, salt, black pepper, coconut cream, and onion. Spread the mixture into the baking sheet.
4. In a small bowl, mix the breadcrumbs with the plant butter and evenly distribute the mixture on top. Add the cheddar cheese and bake the casserole in the oven until golden on top and the cheese melts.
5. Remove the casserole from the oven, allow cooling for 5 minutes, dish, and serve warm.

Nutrition:
Calories 412
Fats 38.14g
Carbs 13.19g
Protein 6.57g

179. Hummus & Vegetable Pizza

Preparation Time: 30 minutes
Serving: 4
If you like hummus, you will LOVE this hummus pizza with mushrooms, spinach and olives.

Ingredients

For the pizza crust:

- 3 ½ cups whole-wheat flour
- 1 tsp yeast
- 1 tsp salt
- 1 pinch sugar
- 3 tbsp olive oil
- 1 cup warm water

For the topping:

- 1 cup hummus
- 10 cremini mushrooms, sliced
- ½ cup fresh baby spinach
- ½ cup cherry tomatoes, halved
- ½ cup sliced Kalamata olives
- ½ medium onion, sliced
- 2 tsp dried oregano

Directions

1. Preheat the oven the 350 F and lightly grease a pizza pan with cooking spray.
2. In a medium bowl, mix the flour, nutritional yeast, salt, sugar, olive oil, and warm water until smooth dough forms. Allow rising for an hour or until the dough doubles in size.
3. Spread the dough on the pizza pan and apply the hummus on the dough. Add the mushrooms, spinach, tomatoes, olives, onion, and top with the oregano. Bake the pizza for 20 minutes or until the mushrooms soften.
4. Remove from the oven, cool for 5 minutes, slice, and serve.

Nutrition:
Calories 592
Fats 19.9g
Carbs 92.5g
Protein 18g

180. Chickpea Burgers With Guacamole

Preparation Time: 20 minutes
Serving: 4
Let's enjoy this burger meatless and it's the perfect time for a guacamole veggie burger!

Ingredients

For the guacamole:

- 1 large avocado, pitted and peeled
- 1 tomato, chopped
- 1 small red onion, chopped

For the burgers:

- 3 (15 ozcans chickpeas, drained and rinsed
- 2 tbsp almond flour
- 2 tbsp quick-cooking oats
- ¼ cup chopped fresh parsley
- 1 tbsp hot sauce
- 1 garlic clove, minced
- ¼ tsp garlic salt
- 1/8 tsp black pepper
- 4 whole-grain hamburger buns, split

Directions

1. In a medium bowl, mash avocados and mix in the tomato, onion, and parsley. Set aside.
2. In a medium bowl, mash the chickpeas and mix in the almond flour, oats, parsley, hot sauce, garlic, garlic salt, and black pepper. Mold 4 patties out of the mixture and set aside.
3. Heat a grill pan to medium heat and lightly grease with cooking spray.

Cooking Time: the bean patties on both sides until light brown and cooked through, 10 minutes. Place each patty between each burger bun and top with the guacamole.

Nutrition:
Calories 369 kcal| Fats 12.7g
Carbs 52.7g
Protein 15.6g

181. Dark Bean And Quinoa Salad With Quick Cumin Dressing

Servings: 4

Ingredients

For the plate of mixed greens:

- 1 cup dry quinoa, washed
- Run salt
- 2 cups vegetable soup or water
- 1/2 huge cucumber, diced conveniently
- 1 little chime pepper, diced conveniently
- 1 can BPA free, natural dark beans
- 10-15 basil leaves, hacked into a chiffonade 1/4 cup crisp cilantro, slashed

For the vinaigrette:

- 2 tbsp additional virgin olive oil
- 1/4 cup apple juice vinegar
- 1 tbsp agave or maple syrup
- 1 tbsp dijon mustard
- 1 tsp cumin
- Salt and pepper to taste

Strategy

1. Rinse quinoa through a strainer till the water runs clear. Move it to a little or medium measured pot and include two cups of vegetable stock or water and run of salt. Heat to the point of

boiling, at that point diminish to a stew. Spread the pot with the goal that the top is on, yet there's a little hole where water can get away. Stew till quinoa has consumed the entirety of the fluid and is soft (around 15-20 minutes).

2. Transfer cooked quinoa to a blending bowl. Include hacked vegetables, dark beans, and herbs.

3. Whisk dressing fixings. Add the dressing to the plate of mixed greens, and serve. (In the event that you don't feel that you need all the dressing, simply include as much as you'd prefer to.

4. Plate of mixed greens will keep for three days in the cooler.

5. Zucchini Pasta With Cherry Tomatoes, Basil, Sweet Potato, And Hemp

182. Hemp Parmesan

Servings: 1/2 - 2/3 cup
Ingredients:

- 6 tbsp hemp seeds
- 6 tbsp dietary yeast
- Run ocean salt

Strategy
Consolidate all fixings in a nourishment processor, and heartbeat to separate and join. Store in the cooler for as long as about fourteen days.

183. Gluten Free White Bean And Summer Vegetable Pasta

Servings: 4
Ingredients:

- 1 little eggplant, cut into 1 inch 3D squares and softly salted for 30 minutes, at that point tapped dry 1 clove garlic, minced

- 1 huge zucchini, cut
- 1 would organic be able to fire simmered, diced tomatoes
- 1 little can natural tomato sauce
- 1 tsp agave
- 1 tbsp dried basil
- 1 tsp dried oregano
- 1 tsp dried thyme
- 1 can (or 2 cups newly cookedcannellini or naval force beans, depleted
- 8 oz. dry dark colored rice or quinoa pasta (rigatoni, linguine, and penne are on the whole fine

Strategy
1. Heat a huge skillet with olive or coconut oil shower (or simply utilize a couple tbsp water). Sautee the eggplant with the garlic till the eggplant is getting decent and darker (around 8 minutes).

2. Add the zucchini and Cooking Time: it till delicate (an additional 5 minutes).

3. Add the canned tomatoes, tomato sauce, agave, basil, oregano, thyme. Warmth through. Test for flavoring, and include a greater amount of whatever herbs you like.

4. Add the white beans and warmth the entire sauce through. This is so delectable and straightforward, you could eat it all alone as a "cheater's" ratatouille.

5. While your sauce cooks, put a pot of salted water to bubble. Include pasta when it hits a moving bubble, and Cooking Time: pasta till delicate yet at the same time somewhat still somewhat firm.

6. Drain pasta, cover with sauce, and serve.

7. Remains will keep for three days in

the ice chest.

184. Butternut Squash Curry

Servings: 4
Ingredients:

- 1 tablespoon dissolved coconut oil
- 1 white or yellow onion, hacked
- 1 clove garlic, minced
- 1 tablespoon new ginger, minced
- 3 tablespoons red curry glue
- 1 tablespoon natural sugar or coconut sugar
- 2/3 cups vegetable soup
- One 14-or 15-ounce would coconut be able to drain
- 1 tablespoon soy sauce or tamari
- 1 green or red chime pepper, slashed
- 1 pound butternut squash
- 2 cups green beans, cut into 2" pieces
- 1 to 2 tablespoon lime juice

Strategy

1. Heat the coconut oil in a huge pot or wok. Include the onion and Cooking Time: till it's delicate and translucent (5 to 8 minutes).
2. Add the garlic and ginger and let them Cooking Time: for about a moment. At that point, include the curry glue and sugar. Combine the fixings until the glue is uniformly consolidated.
3. Whisk in the stock, the coconut milk, and the tamari. Include the red pepper and butternut squash. Stew till the squash is absolutely delicate (25 to 30 minutes). On the off chance that you have to include additional juices as the blend cooks, do as such.
4. Stir in the green beans and let them Cooking Time: for a few minutes, or until delicate. Season the curry to taste with additional soy sauce or tamari

and mix in the lime squeeze as wanted. Expel from warmth and serve over quinoa or darker basmati rice.

5. Remains will keep for four days.

185. Crude Zucchini Alfredo With Basil And Cherry Tomatoes

Servings: 2 (with remaining alfredo sauce
Ingredients:

- Pasta
- 2 huge zucchini
- 1 cup cherry tomatoes, split
- 1/4 cup basil, cut
- Crude alfredo sauce
- 1 cup cashews, drenched for in any event three hours (or medium-termand depleted 1/3 cup water
- 1 tsp agave or maple syrup
- 1 clove garlic
- 3-4 tbsp lemon juice (to taste
- 1/4 cup wholesome yeast
- 1/4 tsp ocean salt

Strategy

1. Use a spiralizer or a julienne peeler to cut zucchini into long strips (looking like noodles).
2. Add tomatoes and basil to the zucchini noodles and put them with or without in an enormous blending bowl.
3. Blend the entirety of the alfredo sauce fixings together in a fast blender till smooth.
4. Cover the pasta in 1/2 cup sauce, and blend it in well, including extra sauce varying (you'll have some sauce remaining). Serve.

186. Dark Bean And Corn Burgers

Servings: 4 Burgers

Ingredients:

- 1 tablespoon coconut oil
- 1 little yellow onion, cleaved
- 1 cup crisp, solidified or canned natural corn pieces
- 1 can natural, low sodium dark beans, depleted (or 1/2 cups cooked dark beans1 cup darker rice, cooked
- 1/4 cup oat flour (or ground, moved oats
- 1/4 cup tomato glue
- 2 tsp cumin
- 1 loading tsp paprika
- 1 loading tsp stew powder
- 1/2 - 1 tsp ocean salt (to taste
- Dark pepper or red pepper, to taste

Technique

1. Preheat your broiler to 350 F.
2. Heat the coconut oil in an enormous sauté dish. Include the onion and saute till onion is brilliant, delicate, and fragrant (around 5-8 minutes).
3. 2Add corn, beans and tomato glue to the container and warmth through.
4. 3Place cooked rice into the bowl of a nourishment processor. Include the beans, onion, tomato glue, and corn blend. Heartbeat to join. Include flavors, oat flour, and a bit of water, on the off chance that you need it. Heartbeat more, until you have a thick and clingy (yet malleableblend. In the event that the blend is excessively wet, include a tablespoon or two of extra oat flour.
5. 4Shape into 4 burgers and spot burgers on a foil lined heating sheet. Prepare for 25 - 30 minutes, or until burgers are delicately crisped, flipping once through. Present with crisp

guacamole, whenever wanted!

187. Eggplant Rollatini With Cashew Cheese

Servings: 4

Ingredients

For rollatini:

- 2 enormous eggplant, cut the long way into 1/4 inch thick cuts
- Olive oil
- 1/4 cups cashews, drenched for in any event three hours (or medium-termand depleted 1/2 tsp ocean salt
- 1 small clove garlic, minced (discretionary
- 2 tbsp lemon juice
- 1/3-1/2 cup water
- 1/4 cup nourishing yeast
- 2 tsps dried basil
- 1 tsp dried oregano
- Dark pepper to taste
- 1/2 10 oz. bundle solidified spinach, defrosted and crushed completely to evacuate all abundance fluid (I press mine immovably through a strainer
- 1/2 cups natural, low sodium marinara sauce

Strategy

1. Preheat stove to 400 F. Cut eggplants the long way into strips around 1/2" thick. Spot eggplant cuts onto heating sheets and sprinkle well with ocean salt or fit salt. Let sit for 30 minutes; this abatements sharpness and expels abundance dampness. Pat the cuts dry, and splash them or brush them gently with olive oil.
2. Roast eggplant cuts till sautéing (around 20 min), flipping part of the way through.
3. While eggplant is cooking, make the

93

cashew cheddar. Spot the cashews, ocean salt, garlic, lemon, and 1/3 cup water in a nourishment processor. Procedure till the blend is extremely smooth and delicate (you're focusing on a surface like velvety ricotta cheddar), halting to scratch the bowl down a couple of times and including some additional water as essential. Stop the engine, and include the wholesome yeast, basil, oregano, and dark pepper. Procedure again to fuse. Move the cashew cheddar to a bowl and blend in the cleaved spinach. Put the cheddar blend in a safe spot.

4. Remove the simmered eggplant from the stove and decrease warmth to 325 F. Permit the cuts to cool until they can be taken care of. Move them to a cutting board and include around 3 tbsp of the cheddar blend as far as possible of one side. Move up from that side, and spot crease down in a little goulash dish. Rehash with every residual cut.

5. Smother the eggplant moves with tomato sauce, and heat, revealed, for around 20-25 minutes, or until hot. Present with sides of decision.

188. Ginger Lime Chickpea Sweet Potato Burgers

Servings: 4-6 Burgers
Ingredients:

- 3/4 cup cooked chickpeas
- 1/2 little onion
- 1 inch ginger, cleaved
- 1 tsp coconut oil
- 1 1/2 cups sweet potato, prepared or steamed and cubed
- 1/3 cup quinoa pieces or gluten free moved oats

- 2 heaping tbsp flax meal
- 2-3 tbsp lime juice (to taste)
- 2 tbsp low sodium tamari
- 1/4 cup cilantro, slashed
- Run red pepper drops (discretionary
- Water varying

Strategy

1. Preheat stove to 350 F.
2. Heat coconut oil in a huge container or wok. Saute onion and ginger in 1 tsp coconut oil (or coconut oil splashtill delicate and fragrant (around 5 minutes). Include chickpeas and warmth through.
3. Place the chickpeas, onion, and ginger in a nourishment processor and include the sweet potato, quinoa chips or oats, flax seed, lime juice, cilantro, tamari or coconut aminos, and run of red pepper drops, if utilizing. Heartbeat to join, at that point run the engine and include some water until consistency is exceptionally thick yet simple to form.
4. Shape blend into 4-6 burgers. Heat at 350 degrees for around 35 minutes, flipping part of the way through.

189. Sweet Potato And Black Bean Chili

Servings: 6
Ingredients:

- 1/2 cup dried dark beans
- 4 cups sweet potato, diced into 3/4 inch solid shapes
- 1 tablespoon olive oil
- 1 1/2 cups slashed white or yellow onion
- 2 cloves garlic, minced
- 1 chipotle pepper en adobo, slashed finely

- 2 teaspoons cumin powder
- 1/2 teaspoon smoked paprika
- 1 tablespoon ground bean stew powder
- 1 14 or 15 ounce container of natural, diced tomatoes (I like the Muir Glen brand
- 1 can natural, low sodium dark beans (or 1/2 cups cooked dark beans2 cups low sodium vegetable soup, Sea salt to taste

Strategy

1. Heat the tablespoon of oil in a dutch stove or a huge pot. Saute the onion for a couple of moments, at that point include the sweet potato and garlic. Keep sauteing until the onions are delicate, around 8-10 minutes.
2. Add the bean stew en adobo, the cumin, the stew powder, and the smoked paprika. Warmth until the flavors are exceptionally fragrant. Include the tomatoes, dark beans, and vegetable soup.
3. When juices is foaming, decrease to a stew and Cooking Time: for roughly 25-30 minutes, or until the sweet potatoes are delicate.
4. Add more juices varying, and season to taste with salt. Serve.
5. Extra stew can be solidified and will keep for as long as five days.

190. Crude Cauliflower Rice With Lemon, Mint, And Pistachios

Servings: 2
Ingredients:

- 5 cups crude cauliflower florets
- 1 oz pistachios
- 1/4 cup every basil and mint
- 2 tsp lemon get-up-and-go

- 1/2 tbsp lemon juice
- 1 tbsp olive oil
- 1/4 cup dried currants
- Ocean Salt And Dark Pepper To Taste

Strategy

1. Transfer 3 cups of the cauliflower to a nourishment processor. Procedure until the cauliflower is separated into pieces that are about the size of rice. Move to a huge blending bowl.
2. Transfer staying 2 cups of cauliflower to the nourishment processor. Include the pistachios. Procedure, by and by, until cauliflower is separated into rice estimated pieces. Heartbeat in the basil and mint till herbs are finely cleaved.
3. Add the extra hacked cauliflower, pistachios, and herbs to the blending bowl in with the principal bunch of cauliflower. Include the lemon juice, oil, and flows. Season to taste with salt and pepper. Serve.

191. Darker Rice And Lentil Salad

Servings: 4
Ingredients:

- 2 tablespoons olive oil
- 1 tablespoon apple juice vinegar
- 1 tablespoon lemon juice
- 1 tablespoon dijon mustard
- 1/2 tsp smoked paprika
- Ocean salt and dark pepper to taste
- 2 cups cooked dark colored rice
- 1 15-oz can natural, no sodium included lentils, flushed, or 1/cups cooked lentils
- 1 carrot, diced or ground
- 4 tbsp cleaved crisp parsley

Technique
1. Whisk oil, vinegar, lemon juice, mustard, paprika, salt and pepper together in a huge bowl.
2. Add the rice, lentils, carrot and parsley. Blend well and serve.

192. Crude "Nut" Noodles

Servings: 2

Ingredients:

For the dressing:

- 1 tablespoon ground ginger
- 1/2 cup olive oil
- 2 tsp sesame oil (toasted
- 2 tbsp smooth white miso
- 3 dates, pitted, or ¼ cup maple syrup
- 1 tbsp nama shoyu
- 1/4 cup water

For the noodles:

- 2 zucchinis
- 1 red chime pepper, cut into matchsticks
- 1 carrot, ground
- 1 little cucumber, stripped into slim strips
- 1 cup daintily cut, steamed snow peas
- 1/4 cup hacked scallions or green onion

Strategy
1. Blend dressing fixings in a rapid blender until all fixings are velvety and smooth.
2. Use a spiralizer or julienne peeler to cut the zucchini into long, slender "noodles." Combine the zucchini with the pepper, carrot, cucumber, and scallions.
3. Dress the noodles with enough dressing to cover them well. Serve.

193. Simple Fried Rice And

Vegetables

Servings: 2

Ingredients:

- 2 tsp toasted sesame oil
- 1 tbsp ground ginger
- 1/2 cups cooked dark colored rice
- 2-3 cups solidified or new vegetables of decision
- 1 tbsp low sodium tamari
- 1 tbsp rice vinegar
- Vegetable Stock Varying

Strategy
1. Heat the sesame oil in a huge wok. Include the ground ginger and warmth it for a moment or two.
2. Add the dark colored rice and vegetables. Saute till the vegetables are delicate.
3. Add the tamari, rice vinegar, and a sprinkle of vegetable soup if the blend is dry. Serve.

194. Arugula Salad With Roasted Butternut Squash, Goji Berries, And Cauliflower

Servings: 2

Ingredients

For the plate of mixed greens:

- 4 piling cups arugula (or other green
- 1 lb butternut squash, stripped and hacked
- 1 small head cauliflower, washed and hacked into little florets
- 2 tbsp coconut or olive oil
- Ocean salt and pepper to taste
- 1/4 cup crude pumpkin seeds
- 1/4 cup goji berries

For the dressing:

- 3 tbsp olive oil
- 2 tbsp squeezed orange

- 1 tbsp lemon juice
- 1/2 tsp turmeric
- 1/4 tsp ground ginger
- 1 tbsp agave or maple syrup
- Ocean salt to taste

Technique

1. Toss the squash in 1 tbsp oil and season with salt and pepper. Hurl the cauliflower in the other tablespoon and season with salt and pepper. Broil the two veggies at 375 degrees for 2030 minutes (the cauliflower will Cooking Time: quicker), till brilliant dark colored and fragrant. Expel from stove and let cool.
2. Place the arugula, goji berries, and pumpkin seeds in an enormous bowl. Include broiled vegetables. Whisk together the olive oil, lemon juice, turmeric, maple syrup or agave, ginger, and ocean salt, and dress all the veggies.
3. Divide serving of mixed greens onto two plates, and serve.

195. Simmered Vegetable Pesto Pasta Salad

Servings: 4
Ingredients:

- 3 cups zucchini, slashed into 3/4" pieces
- 3 cups eggplant, slashed into 3/4" pieces
- 1 large Jersey or legacy tomato, cleaved
- 2 tbsp olive oil or softened coconut oil
- Ocean salt and dark pepper to taste
- 8 oz darker rice or quinoa pasta (penne and fusilli function admirably
- 1/2 - 2/3 cup pecan pesto (see:

dressings

Technique

1. Preheat your broiler to 400 F.
2. Lay the zucchini, eggplant and tomato out on two material or foil fixed heating sheets and shower with the olive or coconut oil. Coat the vegetables with the oil and dish vegetables for thirty minutes, or until delicate and carmelizing.
3. While vegetables cook, carry a pot of salted water to bubble. Include the pasta and Cooking Time: till still somewhat firm (as indicated by bundle directions). Channel pasta and put aside in a huge blending bowl.
4. Add the simmered vegetables and to the pasta. Blend in the pesto, season to taste, and serve on the double.

196. Portobello "Steak" And Cauliflower "Pureed Potatoes"

Servings: 4
Ingredients:

For the mushrooms:

- 1/4 cup olive oil
- 3 tbsp balsamic vinegar
- 3 tbsp low sodium tamari or nama shoyu
- 3 tbsp maple syrup
- Sprinkle pepper
- 4 portobello mushroom tops, cleaned
- Submerge 4 Portobello tops in the marinade. 1 hour will be sufficient for them to be prepared, however medium-term in the refrigerator is far and away superior.

For the Cauliflower Mashed Potatoes:

- 1 cups cashews, crude
- 4 cups cauliflower, slashed into little florets and pieces
- 2 tbsp smooth white miso
- 3 tbsp dietary yeast
- 2 tbsp lemon juice
- Ocean salt and dark pepper to taste
- 1/3 cup (or lesswater

Strategy

1. Place cashews into the bowl of your nourishment processor, and procedure into a fine powder.
2. Add the miso, lemon juice, healthful yeast, pepper and cauliflower. Heartbeat to join. With the engine of the machine running, include water in a flimsy streamin., until the blend starts to take on a smooth, whipped surface. You may need to stop every now and again to clean the sides of the bowl and help it along.
3. When the blend looks like pureed

potatoes, stop, scoop, and serve close by a Portobello top.

197. Quinoa Enchiladas

Adjusted from a formula in Food52
Servings: 6
Ingredients:

- 1 tbsp coconut oil
- 2 cloves garlic, minced
- 1 little yellow onion, cleaved
- 3/4 pounds infant bella mushrooms, hacked
- 1/2 cup diced green bean stews
- 1/2 teaspoon ground cumin
- 1/4 teaspoon ocean salt (or to taste
- 1 can natural, low sodium dark beans or 1/2 cup cooked dark beans
- 1/2 cup cooked quinoa
- 10 6-inch corn tortillas
- 1/4 cup natural, low sodium tomato or enchilada sauce

Technique

1. Preheat broiler to 350 degrees.
2. In an enormous pot over medium warmth, heat coconut oil. Sautee onion and garlic till onion is translucent (around 5-8 min). Include mushrooms and Cooking Time: until fluid has been discharged and vanished (another 5 min).
3. Add the bean stews to the pot and give them a mix for 2 minutes. Include the cumin, ocean salt, dark beans and quinoa, and keep warming the blend until it's totally warm.
4. Spread a flimsy layer (1/2 cupof marinara or enchilada sauce in the base of a goulash dish. Spot 33% of a cup of quinoa blend in the focal point of a corn tortilla and move it up. Spot the tortilla, crease down, in the

goulash dish. Rehash with every outstanding tortilla and afterward spread them with 3/4 cup of extra sauce. Heat for 25 minutes, and serve.

198. Easy Flavored Potatoes Mix

Preparation time: 10 minutes
Cooking time: 25 minutes
Servings: 2
Ingredients:

- 4 potatoes, thinly sliced
- 2 tablespoons olive oil
- 1 fennel bulb, thinly sliced
- 1 tablespoon dill, chopped
- 8 cherry tomatoes, halved
- Salt and black pepper to the taste

Directions:
1. Preheat your air fryer to 365 degrees F and add the oil.
2. Add potato slices, fennel, dill, tomatoes, salt and pepper, toss, cover and Cooking Time: for 25 minutes.
3. Divide potato mix between plates and serve.
4. Enjoy!

Nutrition: calories 240, fat 3, fiber 2, carbs 5, protein 12

199. Eggplant Sandwich

Preparation time: 30 minutes
Cooking time: 30 minutes
Servings: 2
Ingredients:

- 1 eggplant, sliced
- 2 teaspoons parsley, dried
- Salt and black pepper to the taste
- ½ cup vegan breadcrumbs
- ½ teaspoon Italian seasoning
- ½ teaspoon garlic powder
- ½ teaspoon onion powder
- 2 tablespoons almond milk
- 4 vegan bread slices
- Cooking spray
- ½ cup avocado mayo
- ¾ cup tomato sauce
- A handful basil, chopped

Directions:
1. Season eggplant slices with salt and pepper, leave aside for 30 minutes and then pat dry them well.
2. In a bowl, mix parsley with breadcrumbs, Italian seasoning, onion and garlic powder, salt and black pepper and stir.
3. In another bowl, mix milk with vegan mayo and also stir well.
4. Brush eggplant slices with mayo mix, dip them in breadcrumbs mix, place them on a lined baking sheet, spray with cooking oil, introduce baking sheet in your air fryer's basket and Cooking Time: them at 400 degrees F for 15 minutes, flipping them halfway.
5. Brush each bread slice with olive oil and arrange 2 of them on a working surface.
6. Add baked eggplant slices, spread tomato sauce and basil and top with the other bread slices, greased side down.
7. Divide between plates and serve.
8. Enjoy!

Nutrition: calories 324, fat 16, fiber 4, carbs 19, protein 12

200. Veggie Salad

Preparation time: 10 minutes
Cooking time: 15 minutes
Servings: 6
Ingredients:

- 1 green bell pepper, cut into medium chunks

- 1 orange bell pepper, cut into medium chunks
- 1 zucchini, sliced
- 1 red bell pepper, cut into medium chunks
- Salt and black pepper to the taste
- 1 yellow squash, chopped
- 1 red onion, roughly chopped
- 4 ounces brown mushrooms, halved
- 1 teaspoon Italian seasoning
- 1 cups cherry tomatoes, halved
- ½ cup kalamata olives, halved
- 3 tablespoons balsamic vinegar
- 2 tablespoons basil, chopped
- ¼ cup olive oil

Directions:

1. In a bowl, mix all bell peppers with squash, zucchini, mushrooms, onion, half of the olive oil, salt, pepper and Italian seasoning, toss to coat, transfer to the air fryer, Cooking Time: at 380 degrees F for 15 minutes and shake them halfway.
2. In a bowl, mix the veggies with the olives, tomatoes, salt, pepper, vinegar and the rest of the oil, toss to coat and keep in the fridge until you serve.
3. Sprinkle basil on top, divide between plates and serve.
4. Enjoy!

Nutrition: calories 260, fat 8, fiber 4, carbs 14, protein 15

201. Chickpeas Burgers

Preparation time: 10 minutes
Cooking time: 20 minutes
Servings: 2
Ingredients:

- 12 ounces canned chickpeas, drained and mashed
- 2 teaspoons mustard

- Salt and black pepper to the taste
- 3 tablespoons onion, chopped
- 4 teaspoons tomato sauce
- 8 dill pickle chips

Directions:

1. In a bowl, mix chickpeas with salt, pepper, tomato sauce, onion and mustard and stir well.
2. Divide this into 4 pieces, flatten them, top each with dill pickle chips, place burgers in your air fryer's basket and Cooking Time: at 370 degrees F and Cooking Time: for 20 minutes, flipping them after 10 minutes.
3. Divide burgers on vegan buns and serve.
4. Enjoy!

Nutrition: calories 251, fat 5, fiber 7, carbs 12, protein 4

202. Potato Stew

Preparation time: 10 minutes
Cooking time: 25 minutes
Servings: 4
Ingredients:

- 2 carrots, chopped
- 6 potatoes, chopped
- Salt and black pepper to the taste
- 1 quart veggie stock
- ½ teaspoon smoked paprika
- A handful thyme, chopped
- 1 tablespoon parsley, chopped

Directions:

1. In your air fryer, mix carrots, potatoes, stock, salt, pepper, paprika, parsley and thyme, stir and Cooking Time: at 375 degrees F for 25 minutes.
2. Divide into bowls and serve right away.
3. Enjoy!

Nutrition: calories 200, fat 5, fiber 1, carbs 20,

protein 14

203. Greek Veggie Mix

Preparation time: 10 minutes
Cooking time: 20 minutes
Servings: 4
Ingredients:

- A handful cherry tomatoes, halved
- Salt and black pepper to the taste
- 1 parsnip, roughly chopped
- 1 zucchini, roughly chopped
- 1 green bell pepper, cut into strips
- 1 carrot, sliced
- 2 tablespoons stevia
- 1 tablespoon parsley, chopped
- 2 teaspoons garlic, minced
- 6 tablespoons olive oil
- 1 teaspoon mustard

Directions:

1. In your air fryer, mix zucchini with bell pepper, parsnip, carrot, tomatoes, half of the oil, salt and pepper and Cooking Time: at 360 degrees F for 15 minutes.
2. In a bowl, mix the rest of the oil with salt, pepper, stevia, mustard, parsley and garlic and whisk
3. Pour this over veggies, toss to coat, Cooking Time: for 5 minutes more at 375 degrees F, divide between plates and serve.
4. Enjoy!

Nutrition: calories 234, fat 2, fiber 4, carbs 12, protein 7

204. Herbed Mushrooms

Preparation time: 10 minutes
Cooking time: 12 minutes
Servings: 3
Ingredients:

- 10 oyster mushrooms, stems removed
- 1 tablespoon mixed oregano and basil dried
- 1 tablespoon cashew cheese, grated
- A drizzle of olive oil
- 1 tablespoon dill, chopped
- Salt and black pepper to the taste

Directions:

1. Season mushrooms with salt, pepper, mixed herbs, drizzle the oil over them, place them in your air fryer and Cooking Time: at 360 degrees F for 6 minutes.
2. Add cashew cheese and dill, Cooking Time: for 6 minutes more, divide between plates and serve.
3. Enjoy!

Nutrition: calories 210, fat 7, fiber 1, carbs 12, protein 6

205. Corn With Tofu

Preparation time: 10 minutes
Cooking time: 15 minutes
Servings: 4
Ingredients:

- 4 cups corn
- Salt and black pepper to the taste
- 1 tablespoon olive oil
- Juice of 2 limes
- 2 teaspoon smoked paprika
- ½ cup soft tofu, crumbled

Directions:

1. In your air fryer, mix oil with corn, salt, pepper, lime juice and paprika, toss well, cover and Cooking Time: at 400 degrees F for 15 minutes.
2. Divide between plates, sprinkle tofu crumbles all over and serve hot.
3. Enjoy!

Nutrition: calories 160, fat 2, fiber 2, carbs 12, protein 4

206. Garlicky Potatoes

Preparation time: 10 minutes
Cooking time: 40 minutes
Servings: 3
Ingredients:

- 3 big potatoes, peeled and cut into wedges
- Salt and black pepper to the taste
- 2 tablespoons olive oil
- 1 teaspoons sweet paprika
- 2 tablespoons garlic, minced
- 1 tablespoon parsley, chopped

Directions:

1. Put the potatoes in your air fryer's basket, add salt, pepper, garlic, parsley, paprika and oil, toss to coat and Cooking Time: at 392 degrees F for 40 minutes.
2. Divide them between plates and serve hot.
3. Enjoy!

Nutrition: calories 123, fat 1, fiber 2, carbs 21, protein 3

207. Tasty Veggie Mix

Preparation time: 10 minutes
Cooking time: 15 minutes
Servings: 4
Ingredients:

- 2 red onions, cut into chunks
- 2 zucchinis, cut into medium chunks
- 3 tomatoes, cut into wedges
- ¼ cup black olives, pitted and cut into halves
- ¼ cup olive oil
- Salt and black pepper to the taste
- 1 garlic clove, minced
- 1 tablespoon mustard
- 1 tablespoon lemon juice
- ½ cup parsley, chopped

Directions:

1. In your air fryer's pan, mix onion with zucchini, olives, tomatoes, salt, pepper, oil, garlic, mustard and lemon juice, toss, cover and Cooking Time: at 370 degrees F for 15 minutes.
2. Add parsley, toss, divide between plates and serve.
3. Enjoy!

Nutrition: calories 210, fat 1, fiber 4, carbs 7, protein 11

208. French Mushroom Mix

Preparation time: 10 minutes
Cooking time: 25 minutes
Servings: 4
Ingredients:

- 2 pounds mushrooms, halved
- 2 teaspoons herbs de Provence
- ½ teaspoon garlic powder
- 1 tablespoon olive oil

Directions:

1. Heat up a pan with the oil over medium heat, add herbs and heat them up for 2 minutes.
2. Add mushrooms and garlic powder, stir, introduce pan in your air fryer's basket and Cooking Time: at 360 degrees F for 25 minutes.
3. Divide between plates and serve.
4. Enjoy!

Nutrition: calories 152, fat 2, fiber 4, carbs 9, protein 7

209. Easy Broccoli Mix

Preparation time: 10 minutes
Cooking time: 20 minutes
Servings: 4
Ingredients:

- 2 broccoli heads, florets separated
- Juice of ½ lemon
- 1 tablespoon olive oil

- 2 teaspoons sweet paprika
- Salt and black pepper to the taste
- 3 garlic cloves, minced
- 1 tablespoon sesame seeds

Directions:

1. In a bowl, mix broccoli with lemon juice, olive oil, paprika, salt, pepper and garlic, toss to coat, transfer to your air fryer's basket, Cooking Time: at 360 degrees G for 15 minutes, sprinkle sesame seeds, Cooking Time: for 5 minutes more and divide between plates.
2. Serve right away.
3. Enjoy!

Nutrition: calories 156, fat 4, fiber 3, carbs 12, protein 5

210. Zucchini And Squash Salad

Preparation time: 10 minutes
Cooking time: 25 minutes
Servings: 4
Ingredients:

- 6 teaspoons olive oil
- 1 pound zucchinis, cut into half moons
- ½ pound carrots, cubed
- 1 yellow squash, cut into chunks
- Salt and white pepper to the taste
- 1 tablespoon tarragon, chopped
- 2 tablespoons tomato paste

Directions:

1. In your air fryer's pan, mix oil with zucchinis, carrots, squash, salt, pepper, tarragon and tomato paste, cover and Cooking Time: at 400 degrees F for 25 minutes.
2. Divide between plates and serve.
3. Enjoy!

Nutrition: calories 170, fat 2, fiber 2, carbs 12, protein 5

211. Indian Cauliflower Mix

Preparation time: 10 minutes
Cooking time: 20 minutes
Servings: 4
Ingredients:

- 3 cups cauliflower florets
- Salt and black pepper to the taste
- A drizzle of olive oil
- ½ cup veggie stock
- ¼ teaspoon turmeric powder
- 1 and ½ teaspoon red chili powder
- 1 tablespoon ginger paste
- 2 teaspoons lemon juice
- 2 tablespoons water

Directions:

1. In your air fryer's pan, mix stock with cauliflower, oil, salt, pepper, turmeric, chili powder, ginger paste, lemon juice and water, stir, cover and Cooking Time: at 400 degrees F for 10 minutes and at 360 degrees F for another 10 minutes.
2. Divide between bowls and serve.
3. Enjoy!

Nutrition: calories 150, fat 1, fiber 2, carbs 12, protein 3

212. "Baked" Potatoes

Preparation time: 10 minutes
Cooking time: 40 minutes
Servings: 3
Ingredients:

- 3 big baking potatoes
- 1 teaspoon dill, chopped
- 1 tablespoon garlic, minced
- Salt and black pepper to the taste
- 2 tablespoons olive oil

Directions:

1. Prick potatoes with a fork, season with salt and pepper to the taste, rub

with the oil, garlic and dill, place them in your air fryer's basket and Cooking Time: at 392 degrees F for 40 minutes.

2. Divide them between plates and serve.
3. Enjoy!

Nutrition: calories 130, fat 2, fiber 3, carbs 23, protein 4

SIDES AND SALADS

213. Squash & Pomegranate Salad

Preparation time: 10 minutes
Cooking time: 0 minutes
Total time: 10 minutes
Servings: 04
Ingredients:

Vegetables:

- 5 cups butternut squash, boiled, peeled, and cubed
- 1 tablespoon coconut oil, melted
- 1 tablespoon coconut sugar
- 1 pinch cayenne pepper
- 1 healthy pinch salt
- ½ teaspoon ground cinnamon
- 2 tablespoons maple syrup

Nuts:

- 1 cup raw pecans
- 2 teaspoons coconut oil
- 1 tablespoon maple syrup
- 1 tablespoon coconut sugar
- 1 pinch cayenne pepper
- 1 pinch salt
- ½ teaspoon ground cinnamon

Pomegranate Dressing:

- ¼ cup pomegranate molasses
- 2 cups mixed greens
- Juice from ½ a medium lemon
- 2 teaspoons olive oil
- 1 pinch salt
- Black pepper, to taste
- ½ cup pomegranate arils
- ¼ cup red onion, sliced

How to Prepare:

1. In a salad bowl, add butternut cubes and all the salad ingredients.
2. In a separate bowl, toss all the nuts together.
3. Prepare the dressing by mixing all the dressing ingredients in a different bowl.
4. Add nuts and dressing to the squash and mix well.
5. Serve.

Nutritional Values:
Calories 210.6
Total Fat 10.91 g
Saturated Fat 7.4 g
Sodium 875 mg
Potassium 604 mg
Carbohydrates 25.6 g
Fiber 4.3 g
Sugar 7.9 g
Protein 2.1 g

214. French Style Potato Salad

Preparation time: 10 minutes
Cooking time: 0 minutes
Total time: 10 minutes
Servings: 04
Ingredients:

Potatoes:

- 2 pounds baby yellow potatoes, boiled, peeled, and diced
- 1 pinch salt and black pepper
- 1 tablespoon apple cider vinegar
- 1 cup green onion, diced
- ¼ cup fresh parsley, chopped

Dressing:

- 2½ tablespoons brown mustard
- 3 cloves garlic, minced
- ¼ teaspoon salt and black pepper
- 3 tablespoons red wine vinegar
- 1 tablespoon apple cider vinegar
- 3 tablespoons olive oil

- ¼ cup dill, chopped

How to Prepare:
1. Combine all the dressing ingredients in a salad bowl.
2. In a salad bowl, toss in all the vegetables, seasonings, and dressing.
3. Mix them well then refrigerate to chill.
4. Serve.

Nutritional Values:
Calories 197
Total Fat 4 g
Saturated Fat 0.5 g
Cholesterol 135 mg
Sodium 790 mg
Total Carbs 31 g
Fiber 12.2 g
Sugar 2.5 g
Protein 11 g

215. Mango Salad With Peanut Dressing

Preparation time: 10 minutes
Cooking time: 0 minutes
Total time: 10 minutes
Servings: 04
Ingredients:

Salad:
- 1 head butter lettuce, washed and chopped
- 1½ cups carrot, shredded
- 1¼ cups red cabbage, shredded
- 1 large ripe mango, cubed
- ½ cup fresh cilantro, chopped

Dressing:
- ⅓ cup creamy peanut butter
- 2½ tablespoons lime juice
- 1½ tablespoons maple syrup
- 2 teaspoon chili garlic sauce
- 3 tablespoons coconut aminos

How to Prepare:

1. Combine all the dressing ingredients in a small bowl.
2. In a salad bowl, toss in all the vegetables, seasonings, and dressing.
3. Mix them well then refrigerate to chill.
4. Serve.

Nutritional Values:
Calories 305
Total Fat 11.8 g
Saturated Fat 2.2 g
Cholesterol 56 mg
Sodium 321 mg
Total Carbs 34.6 g
Fibers 0.4 g
Sugar 2 g
Protein 7 g

216. Loaded Kale Salad

Preparation time: 10 minutes
Cooking time: 0 minutes
Total time: 10 minutes
Servings: 04
Ingredients:

Quinoa:
- ¾ cups quinoa, cooked and drained

Vegetables:
- 4 large carrots, halved and chopped
- 1 whole beet, sliced
- 2 tablespoons water
- 1 pinch salt
- ½ teaspoon curry powder
- 8 cups kale, chopped
- ½ cups cherry tomatoes, chopped
- 1 ripe avocado, cubed
- ¼ cup hemp seeds
- ½ cup sprouts

Dressing:
- ⅓ cup tahini
- 3 tablespoons lemon juice
- 1-2 tablespoons maple syrup

- 1 pinch salt
- ¼ cup water

How to Prepare:
1. Combine all the dressing ingredients in a small bowl.
2. In a salad bowl, toss in all the vegetables, quinoa, and dressing.
3. Mix them well then refrigerate to chill.
4. Serve.

Nutritional Values:
Calories 72
Total Fat 15.4 g
Saturated Fat 4.2 g
Cholesterol 168 mg
Sodium 203 mg
Total Carbs 28.5 g
Sugar 1.1 g
Fiber 4 g
Protein 7.9 g

217. Cauliflower & Lentil Salad

Preparation time: 10 minutes
Cooking time: 25 minutes
Total time: 35 minutes
Servings: 04
Ingredients:

Cauliflower:
- 1 head cauliflower, florets
- 1½ tablespoons melted coconut oil
- 1½ tablespoons curry powder
- ¼ teaspoon salt

Salad:
- 5 cups mixed greens
- 1 cup cooked lentils
- 1 cup red or green grapes, halved
- Fresh cilantro

Tahini Dressing:
- 4½ tablespoons green curry paste
- 2 tablespoons tahini
- 2 tablespoons lemon juice

- 1 tablespoon maple syrup
- 1 pinch salt
- 1 pinch black pepper
- Water to thin

How to Prepare:
1. Preheat your oven to 400 degrees F.
2. On a greased baking sheet, toss cauliflower with salt, curry powder, and oil.
3. Bake the cauliflower for 25 minutes in the oven.
4. Combine all the dressing ingredients in a small bowl.
5. In a salad bowl, toss in all the vegetables, roasted cauliflower, and dressing.
6. Mix them well then refrigerate to chill.
7. Serve.

Nutritional Values:
Calories 212
Total Fat 7 g
Saturated Fat 1.3 g
Cholesterol 25 mg
Sodium 101 mg
Total Carbs 32.5 g
Sugar 5.7 g
Fiber 6 g
Protein 4 g

218. Sweet Potato & Avocado Salad

Preparation time: 10 minutes
Cooking time: 20 minutes
Total time: 30 minutes
Servings: 50
Ingredients:

Sweet potato:
- 1 large organic sweet potato, cubed
- 1 tablespoon avocado or coconut oil
- 1 pinch salt

Dressing:

- ¼ cup tahini
- 2 tablespoons lemon juice
- 1 tablespoon maple syrup
- 1 pinch salt
- Water

Salad:

- 5 cups greens of choice
- 1 medium ripe avocado, chopped
- 2 tablespoons hemp seeds

How to Prepare:

1. Preheat your oven to 375 degrees.
2. On a greased baking sheet, toss sweet potato with salt and oil.
3. Bake the potatoes for 20 minutes in the oven, toss halfway through.
4. Combine all the dressing ingredients in a small bowl.
5. In a salad bowl, toss in all the vegetables, roasted potato, and dressing.
6. Mix them well then refrigerate to chill.
7. Serve.

Nutritional Values:

Calories 119

Total Fat 14 g

Saturated Fat 2 g

Cholesterol 65 mg

Sodium 269 mg

Total Carbs 19 g

Fiber 4 g

Sugar 6 g

Protein 5g

219. Broccoli Sweet Potato Chickpea Salad

Preparation time: 10 minutes

Cooking time: 22 minutes

Total time: 32 minutes

Servings: 06

Ingredients:

Vegetables:

- 1 large sweet potato, peeled and diced
- 1 head broccoli
- 2 tablespoons olive or grapeseed oil
- 1 pinch each salt and black pepper
- 1 teaspoon dried dill
- 1 medium red bell pepper

Chickpeas:

- 1 (15 ouncecan chickpeas, drained
- 1 tablespoon olive or grapeseed oil
- 1 tablespoon tandoori masala spice
- 1 pinch salt
- 1 teaspoon coconut sugar
- 1 pinch cayenne pepper

Garlic dill sauce:

- ⅓ cup hummus
- 3 large cloves garlic, minced
- 1 teaspoon dried dill
- 2 tablespoons lemon juice
- Water

How to Prepare:

1. Preheat your oven to 400 degrees F.
2. In a greased baking sheet, toss sweet potato with salt and oil.
3. Bake the sweet potatoes for 15 minutes in the oven.
4. Toss all chickpea ingredients and spread in a tray.
5. Bake them for 7 minutes in the oven.
6. Combine all the sauce ingredients in a small bowl.
7. In a salad bowl, toss in all the vegetables, roasted potato, chickpeas, and sauce.
8. Mix them well then refrigerate to chill.
9. Serve.

Nutritional Values:

Calories 231

Total Fat 20.1 g

Saturated Fat 2.4 g

Cholesterol 110 mg
Sodium 941 mg
Total Carbs 20.1 g
Fiber 0.9 g
Sugar 1.4 g
Protein 4.6 g

220. Penne Pasta Salad

Preparation time: 30 minutes
Cooking time: 0 minutes
Total time: 30 minutes
Servings: 04
Ingredients:
Salad:

- 2 cups roasted tomatoes
- 12 ounces penne pasta

Pesto:

- 2 cups fresh basil
- 4 cloves garlic, minced
- ¼ cup toasted pine nuts
- 1 medium lemon, juice
- ¼ cup vegan cheese, shredded
- 1 pinch salt
- ¼ cup olive oil

How to Prepare:
1. In a blender, add all the pesto ingredients.
2. Blend them well until it is lump free.
3. In a salad bowl toss in pasta, roasted tomatoes, and pesto.
4. Mix them well then refrigerate to chill.
5. Serve.

Nutritional Values:
Calories 361
Total Fat 16.3 g
Saturated Fat 4.9 g
Cholesterol 114 mg
Sodium 515 mg
Total Carbs 29.3 g
Fiber 0.1 g

Sugar 18.2 g
Protein 3.3 g

221. Roasted Fennel Salad

Preparation time: 10 minutes
Cooking time: 20 minutes
Total time: 30 minutes
Servings: 4
Ingredients:
Fennel:

- 1 bulb fennel fronds, sliced
- 1 tablespoon curry powder
- 1 tablespoon avocado oil
- 1 pinch salt

Salad:

- 5 cups salad greens
- 1 red bell pepper, sliced

Dressing:

- ¼ cup tahini
- 1½ tablespoons lemon juice
- 1½ teaspoons apple cider vinegar
- 1 tablespoon freshly minced rosemary
- 3 cloves garlic, minced
- 1½ tablespoons coconut aminos
- 5 tablespoons water to thin
- 1 pinch salt

How to Prepare:
1. Preheat your oven at 375 degrees F.
2. On a greased baking sheet, toss fennel with salt, curry powder, and oil.
3. Bake the curried fennel for 20 minutes in the oven.
4. Combine all the dressing ingredients in a small bowl.
5. In a salad bowl, toss in all the vegetables, roasted fennel, and dressing.
6. Mix them well then refrigerate to chill.
7. Serve.

Nutritional Values:
Calories 205
Total Fat 22.7 g
Saturated Fat 6.1 g
Cholesterol 4 mg
Sodium 227 mg
Total Carbs 26.1 g
Fiber 1.4 g
Sugar 0.9 g
Protein 5.2 g

222. Kale Salad With Tahini Dressing

Preparation time: 10 minutes
Cooking time: 20 minutes
Total time: 30 minutes
Servings: 04
Ingredients:

Roasted vegetables:
- 1 medium zucchini, chopped
- 1 medium sweet potato, chopped
- 1 cup red cabbage, chopped
- 1 tablespoon melted coconut oil
- 1 pinch salt
- ½ teaspoon curry powder

Dressing:
- ⅓ cup tahini
- ½ teaspoon garlic powder
- 1 tablespoon coconut aminos
- 1 pinch salt
- 1 large clove garlic, minced
- ¼ cup water

Salad:
- 6 cups mixed greens
- 4 small radishes, sliced
- 3 tablespoons hemp seeds
- 2 tablespoons lemon juice
- ½ ripe avocado, to garnish
- 2 tablespoons vegan feta cheese, crumbled
- Pomegranate seeds, to garnish
- Pecans, to garnish

How to Prepare:
1. Preheat your oven at 375 degrees F.
2. On a greased baking sheet, toss zucchini, sweet potato, and red cabbage with salt, curry powder, and oil.
3. Bake the zucchini cabbage mixture for 20 minutes in the oven.
4. Combine all the dressing ingredients in a small bowl.
5. In a salad bowl, toss in all the vegetables, roasted vegetables, and dressing.
6. Mix them well then refrigerate to chill.
7. Garnish with feta cheese, pecans, pomegranate seeds and avocado.
8. Serve.

Nutritional Values:
Calories 201
Total Fat 8.9 g
Saturated Fat 4.5 g
Cholesterol 57 mg
Sodium 340 mg
Total Carbs 24.7 g
Fiber 1.2 g
Sugar 1.3 g
Protein 15.3 g

223. Roasted Squash Salad

Preparation time: 10 minutes
Cooking time: 20 minutes
Total time: 30 minutes
Servings: 04
Ingredients:
Squash:
- 1 medium acorn squash, peeled and cubed
- 1 tablespoon avocado oil

- 1 pinch each salt and black pepper

Dressing:
- 1 cup balsamic vinegar

Salad:
- ¼ cup macadamia nut cheese
- 2 tablespoons roasted pumpkin seeds
- 5 cups arugula
- 2 tablespoons dried currants

How to Prepare:
1. Preheat your oven to 425 degrees F.
2. On a greased baking sheet, toss squash with salt, black pepper, and oil.
3. Bake the seasoned squash for 20 minutes in the oven.
4. Combine all the dressing ingredients in a small bowl.
5. In a salad bowl, toss in the squash, salad ingredients, and dressing.
6. Mix them well then refrigerate to chill.
7. Serve.

Nutritional Values:
Calories 119
Total Fat 14 g
Saturated Fat 2 g
Cholesterol 65 mg
Sodium 269 mg
Total Carbs 19 g
Fiber 4 g
Sugar 6 g
Protein 5g

224. Vegetable Salad With Chimichurri

Preparation time: 10 minutes
Cooking time: 25 minutes
Total time: 35 minutes
Servings: 04
Ingredients:

Roasted vegetables:
- 1 large sweet potato (chopped
- 6 red potatoes, quartered
- 2 whole carrots, chopped
- 2 tablespoons melted coconut oil
- 2 teaspoons curry powder
- ½ teaspoon salt
- 1 cup chopped broccolini
- 2 cups red cabbage, chopped
- 1 medium red bell pepper, sliced

Chimichurri:
- 5 cloves garlic, chopped
- 1 medium serrano pepper
- 1 cup packed cilantro
- 1 cup parsley
- 3 tablespoons ripe avocado
- ¼ teaspoon salt
- 3 tablespoons lime juice
- 1 tablespoon maple syrup
- Water to thin

Salad:
- 4 cups hearty greens
- 1 medium ripe avocado, chopped
- 3 tablespoons hemp seeds
- Fresh herbs
- 5 medium radishes, sliced
- ¼ cup macadamia nut cheese

How to Prepare:
1. Preheat your oven to 400 degrees F.
2. In a suitable bowl, toss all the vegetables for roasting with salt, curry powder and oil.
3. Divide these vegetables into two roasting pans.
4. Bake the vegetables for 25 minutes in the oven.
5. Meanwhile, in a blender, blend all chimichurri sauce ingredients until smooth.
6. In a salad bowl, toss in all the roasted vegetables, chimichurri sauce and salad ingredients.

7. Mix them well then refrigerate to chill.
8. Serve.

Nutritional Values:
Calories 231
Total Fat 20.1 g
Saturated Fat 2.4 g
Cholesterol 110 mg
Sodium 941 mg
Total Carbs 20.1 g
Fiber 0.9 g
Sugar 1.4 g
Protein 4.6 g

225. Thai Salad With Tempeh

Preparation time: 10 minutes
Cooking time: 0 minutes
Total time: 10 minutes
Servings: 04
Ingredients:
Salad:

- 6 ounces vermicelli noodles, boiled
- 2 medium whole carrots, ribboned
- 2 stalks green onions, chopped
- ¼ cup cilantro, chopped
- 2 tablespoons mint, chopped
- 1 cup packed spinach, chopped
- 1 cup red cabbage, sliced
- 1 medium red bell pepper, sliced

Dressing:

- ⅓ cup creamy peanut butter
- 3 tablespoons tamari
- 3 tablespoons maple syrup
- 1 teaspoon chili garlic sauce
- 1 medium lime, juiced
- ¼ cup water

How to Prepare:
1. Combine all the dressing ingredients in a small bowl.
2. In a salad bowl, toss in the noodles, salad, and dressing.

3. Mix them well then refrigerate to chill.
4. Serve.

Nutritional Values:
Calories 361
Total Fat 16.3 g
Saturated Fat 4.9 g
Cholesterol 114 mg
Sodium 515 mg
Total Carbs 29.3 g
Fiber 0.1 g
Sugar 18.2 g
Protein 3.3 g

226. Niçoise Salad

Preparation time: 10 minutes
Cooking time: 15 minutes
Total time: 25 minutes
Servings: 04
Ingredients:
Salad:

- 6 small red potatoes, peeled, boiled, and diced
- 1 cup green beans, chopped
- 1 head lettuce, chopped
- ½ cup pitted kalamata olives
- ½ cup tomato, sliced
- ½medium red beet

Chickpeas:

- 1 (15 ouncecan chickpeas
- 1 teaspoon Dijon mustard
- 1 teaspoon maple syrup
- 1 teaspoon dried dill
- 1 pinch salt
- 1 tablespoon roasted sunflower seeds

Dressing:

- 3 tablespoons minced shallot
- 1 heaping teaspoon Dijon mustard
- 1 teaspoon fresh thyme, chopped
- ⅓ cup red wine vinegar

- ¼ teaspoon salt and black pepper
- ¼ cup olive oil

How to Prepare:
1. Preheat your oven to 400 degrees F.
2. In a greased baking sheet, toss chickpeas with salt and all the chickpea ingredients.
3. Bake the chickpeas for 15 minutes in the oven.
4. Combine all the dressing ingredients in a small bowl.
5. In a salad bowl, toss in all the vegetables, roasted chickpeas, and dressing.
6. Mix them well then refrigerate to chill.
7. Serve.

Nutritional Values:
Calories 205
Total Fat 22.7 g
Saturated Fat 6.1 g
Cholesterol 4 mg
Sodium 227 mg
Total Carbs 26.1 g
Fiber 1.4 g
Sugar 0.9 g
Protein 5.2 g

227. Avocado Kale Salad

Preparation time: 10 minutes
Cooking time: 0 minutes
Total time: 10 minutes
Servings: 04
Ingredients:

Dressing:
- ⅓ cup tahini
- 2 teaspoons garlic, chopped
- 1 medium lemon juiced
- 1½ tablespoons maple syrup
- Water

Salad:

- 1 large bundle kale, chopped
- 1 tablespoon grapeseed oil
- 1 tablespoon lemon juice
- 1 medium beet

How to Prepare:
1. Combine all the dressing ingredients in a small bowl.
2. In a salad bowl, toss in all the salad ingredients and dressing.
3. Mix them well then refrigerate to chill.
4. Serve.

Nutritional Values:
Calories 201
Total Fat 8.9 g
Saturated Fat 4.5 g
Cholesterol 57 mg
Sodium 340 mg
Total Carbs 24.7 g
Fiber 1.2 g
Sugar 1.3 g
Protein 15.3 g

228. Sesame Seed Simple Mix

Preparation Time: 5minutes
Servings: 2

Ingredients
- Frozen peas: 1 cup can washed and drained
- Corn kernel: 2 cups can
- Salt: as per your taste
- Sesame seeds: 2 tbsp
- Pepper: as per your taste
- Cashew cream: ½ cup

Directions:
1. Combine all the ingredients
2. Serve as the side dish

Nutrition:
Carbs: 44.5g
Protein: 11.5g
Fats: 11.4g
Calories: 306Kcal

229. Cherry Tomato Salad With Soy Chorizo

Preparation Time: 5 minutes
Cooking Time: 5 minutes
Serving Size: 4
Ingredients:

- 2 ½ tbsp olive oil
- 4 soy chorizo, chopped
- 2 tsp red wine vinegar
- 1 small red onion, finely chopped
- 2 ½ cups cherry tomatoes, halved
- 2 tbsp chopped cilantro
- Salt and freshly ground black pepper to taste
- 3 tbsp sliced black olives to garnish

Directions:

1. Over medium fire, heat half tablespoon of olive oil in a skillet and fry soy chorizo until golden. Turn heat off.
2. In a salad bowl, whisk remaining olive oil and vinegar. Add onion, cilantro, tomatoes, and soy chorizo. Mix with dressing and season with salt and black pepper.
3. Garnish with olives and serve.

Nutrition:
Calories 138, Total Fat 8.95g, Total Carbs 5.63g, Fiber 0.4g, Net Carbs 5.23g, Protein 7.12g

230. Roasted Bell Pepper Salad With Olives

Preparation Time: 10 minutes
Cooking Time: 20 minutes
Serving Size: 4
Ingredients:

- 8 large red bell peppers, deseeded and cut in wedges
- ½ tsp erythritol
- 2 ½ tbsp olive oil
- 1/3 cup arugula
- 1 tbsp mint leaves
- 1/3 cup pitted Kalamata olives
- 3 tbsp chopped almonds
- ½ tbsp balsamic vinegar
- Crumbled feta cheese for topping
- Toasted pine nuts for topping

Directions:

1. Preheat oven to 400o F.
2. Pour bell peppers on a roasting pan; season with erythritol and drizzle with half of olive oil. Roast in oven until slightly charred, 20 minutes. Remove from oven and set aside.
3. Arrange arugula in a salad bowl, scatter bell peppers on top, mint leaves, olives, almonds, and drizzle with balsamic vinegar and remaining olive oil. Season with salt and black pepper.
4. Toss; top with feta cheese and pine nuts and serve.

Nutrition:
Calories 163, Total Fat 13.3g, Total Carbs 6.53g, Fiber 2.2g, Net Carbs 4.33g, Protein 3.37g

231. Tofu-Dulse-Walnut Salad

Preparation Time: 10 minutes
Cooking Time: 15 minutes
Serving Size: 4
Ingredients:

- 1 (7 ozblock extra firm tofu
- 2 tbsp olive oil
- 2 tbsp butter
- 1 cup asparagus, trimmed and halved
- 1 cup green beans, trimmed
- 2 tbsp chopped dulse
- Salt and freshly ground black pepper to taste

- ½ lemon, juiced
- 4 tbsp chopped walnuts

Directions:

1. Place tofu in between two paper towels and allow soaking for 5 minutes. After, remove towels and chop into small cubes.
2. Heat olive oil in a skillet and fry tofu until golden, 10 minutes. Remove onto a paper towel-lined plate and set aside.
3. Melt butter in skillet and sauté asparagus and green beans until softened, 5 minutes. Add dulse, season with salt and black pepper, and Cooking Time: until softened. Mix in tofu and stir-fry for 5 minutes.
4. Plate, drizzle with lemon juice, and scatter walnuts on top.
5. Serve warm.

Nutrition:

Calories 237, Total Fat 19.57g, Total Carbs 5.9g, Fiber 2.1g, Net Carbs 3.89, Protein 12.75g

232. Almond-Goji Berry Cauliflower Salad

Preparation Time: 10 minutes
Cooking Time: 2 minutes
Serving Size: 4
Ingredients:

- 1 small head cauliflower, cut into florets
- 8 sun-dried tomatoes in olive oil, drained
- 12 pitted green olives, roughly chopped
- 1 lemon, zested and juiced
- 3 tbsp chopped green onions
- A handful chopped almonds
- ¼ cup goji berries

- 1 tbsp sesame oil
- ½ cup watercress
- 3 tbsp chopped parsley
- Salt and freshly ground black pepper to taste
- Lemon wedges to garnish

Directions:

1. Pour cauliflower into a large safe-microwave bowl, sprinkle with some water, and steam in microwave for 1 to 2 minutes or until softened.
2. In a large salad bowl, combine cauliflower, tomatoes, olives, lemon zest and juice, green onions, almonds, goji berries, sesame oil, watercress, and parsley. Season with salt and black pepper, and mix well.
3. Serve with lemon wedges.

Nutrition:

Calories 203, Total Fat 15.28g, Total Carbs 9.64g, Fiber 3.2g, Net Carbs 6.44g, Protein 6.67g, Protein 2.54g

233. Warm Mushroom And Orange Pepper Salad

Preparation Time: 10 minutes
Cooking Time: 8 minutes
Serving Size: 4
Ingredients:

- 2 tbsp avocado oil
- 1 cup mixed mushrooms, chopped
- 2 orange bell peppers, deseeded and finely sliced
- 1 garlic clove, minced
- 2 tbsp tamarind sauce
- 1 tsp maple (sugar-freesyrup
- ½ tsp hot sauce
- ½ tsp fresh ginger paste
- Sesame seeds to garnish

Directions:

1. Over medium fire, heat half of

115

avocado oil in a large skillet, sauté mushroom and bell peppers until slightly softened, 5 minutes.

2. In a small bowl, whisk garlic, tamarind sauce, maple syrup, hot sauce, and ginger paste. Add mixture to vegetables and stir-fry for 2 to 3 minutes.
3. Turn heat off and dish salad. Drizzle with remaining avocado oil and garnish with sesame seeds.
4. Serve with grilled tofu.

Nutrition:
Calories 289, Total Fat 26.71g, Total Carbs 9g, Fiber 3.8g, Net Carbs 5.2g, Protein 4.23g

234. Broccoli, Kelp, And Feta Salad

Preparation Time: 15 minutes
Serving Size: 4
Ingredients:

- 2 tbsp olive oil
- 1 tbsp white wine vinegar
- 2 tbsp chia seeds
- Salt and freshly ground black pepper to taste
- 2 cups broccoli slaw
- 1 cup chopped kelp, thoroughly washed and steamed
- 1/3 cup chopped pecans
- 1/3 cup pumpkin seeds
- 1/3 cup blueberries
- 2/3 cup ricotta cheese

Directions:

1. In a small bowl, whisk olive oil, white wine vinegar, chia seeds, salt, and black pepper. Set aside.
2. In a large salad bowl, combine the broccoli slaw, kelp, pecans, pumpkin seeds, blueberries, and ricotta cheese.
3. Drizzle dressing on top, toss, and serve.

Nutrition:
Calories 397, Total Fat 3.87g, Total Carbs 8.4g, Fiber 3.5g, Net Carbs 4.9g, Protein 8.93g

235. Roasted Asparagus With Feta Cheese Salad

Preparation Time: 10 minutes
Cooking Time: 20 minutes
Serving Size: 4
Ingredients:

- 1 lb asparagus, trimmed and halved
- 2 tbsp olive oil
- ½ tsp dried basil
- ½ tsp dried oregano
- Salt and freshly ground black pepper to taste
- ½ tsp hemp seeds
- 1 tbsp maple (sugar-freesyrup
- ½ cup arugula
- 4 tbsp crumbled feta cheese
- 2 tbsp hazelnuts
- 1 lemon, cut into wedges

Directions:

1. Preheat oven to 350oF.
2. Pour asparagus on a baking tray, drizzle with olive oil, basil, oregano, salt, black pepper, and hemp seeds. Mix with your hands and roast in oven for 15 minutes.
3. Remove, drizzle with maple syrup, and continue cooking until slightly charred, 5 minutes.
4. Spread arugula in a salad bowl and top with asparagus. Scatter with feta cheese, hazelnuts, and serve with lemon wedges.

Nutrition:
Calories 146, Total Fat 12.87g, Total Carbs 5.07g, Fiber 1.6g, Net Carbs 3.47g, Protein 4.44g

236. Spicy Avocado Bites

Preparation Time: 25 minutes
Servings: 4

Ingredients

- Avocado mashed:1
- Cucumbers:2cut into thick slices
- Lemon: 1 tsp
- Salt and pepper: as per your taste
- Vegan chipotle mayo:2 tbsp
- Spicy roasted chickpeas:½ pack
- Fresh herbs:3 tbsp

Directions:
1. Add lemon and seasoning to the mashed avocado
2. Place on each cucumber slice and press using chickpeas
3. Top with herbs and mayo and serve

Nutrition:
Carbs: 5 g
Protein: 1 g
Fats: 10 g
Calories: 110 Kcal

237. Spicy Broccoli Salad

Preparation Time: 45 minutes
Servings: 2

Ingredients

- Broccoli: 2 cups cut in big florets
- Hot sauce: 2 tbsp
- Rice vinegar: 1 tbsp
- Salt: as per your taste
- Pepper: as per your taste
- Sliced red pepper: 1 cup sliced
- Olive oil: 1 tbsp

Directions:
1. Preheat the oven 200C
2. Add broccoli to the baking sheet and sprinkle seasoning and brush with olive oil
3. Roast for 25 minutes till it turns golden and soft
4. Take a small bowl and combine hot sauce, vinegar, salt, and pepper
5. Remove broccoli from oven and brush with this dressing and Cooking Time: in the oven again for 10 minutes
6. Add to the serving bowl and serve with red pepper
7. Serve as the side dish

Nutrition:
Carbs: 10.5 g
Protein:2.6g
Fats: 7.5g
Calories: 133Kcal

238. Spinach Hummus

Preparation Time: 10 minutes
Servings: 4 as a side dish

Ingredients

- Chickpeas: 2 cups tin drained and rinsed
- Baby spinach: 1 cup
- Tahini: 3 tbsp
- Garlic: 1 clove
- Lemon: 2 tbsp
- Extra-virgin olive oil: 3 tbsp, plus extra to serve
- Salt: as per your need

Directions:
- Blend baby spinach, chickpeas, tahini, olive oil, salt, and garlic together in a blender
- Add in lemon juice and mix
- Add to the serving bowl and top with extra olive oil

Nutrition:
Carbs: 25.8g
Protein: 10.7g
Fats: 18.6g
Calories: 296Kcal

239. Stir Fry Turmeric Butternut Squash

Preparation Time: 30 minutes
Servings: 2

Ingredients

- Olive oil: 2 tbsp
- Butternut squash: 2 cups
- Turmeric: 1 tsp
- Salt: as per your taste
- Red pepper: ½ tsp

Directions:

1. Take a pan and heat olive oil
2. Take a bowl and add butternut squash, salt, turmeric, pepper and mix well and add to the pan
3. Fry on low heat for 20 minutes and turn in between
4. Serve as a salad with the main dish

Nutrition:
Carbs: 22g
Protein:1.9g
Fats:14.2g
Calories: 201Kcal

240. Rainbow Vegetable Bowl

Preparation Time: 25 minute
Servings: 4

Ingredients

- Red bell Pepper: 1
- Yellow bell pepper: 1
- Smoked Paprika: ½ tsp
- Potatoes: 3 medium
- Mushrooms: 8 oz
- Yellow Onion: 1
- Zucchini: 1
- Cumin Powder: ½ tsp
- Garlic Powder: ½ tsp
- Salt and Pepper: as per your taste
- Cooking oil: 2 tbsp (optional

Directions:

1. Heat a large pan on medium flame, add oil and put the sliced potatoes
2. Cooking Time: the potatoes till they change color
3. Cut the rest of the vegetables and add all the spices
4. Cooked till veggies are soften

Nutrition:
Carbs: 29.9g
Protein: 5.9g
Fats: 10g
Calories: 227 Kcal

241. Red Bell Pepper Hummus

Preparation Time: 10 minutes
Servings: 4 as a side dish

Ingredients

- Chickpeas: 2 cups can rinsed and drained
- Red bell pepper: 1 cup diced
- Tahini: 3 tbsp
- Garlic: 1 clove
- Lemon: 2 tbsp
- Extra-virgin olive oil: 3 tbsp, plus extra to serve
- Salt: as per your need
- Cayenne pepper: 1 tsp

Directions:

1. Blend red bell pepper, chickpeas, tahini, olive oil, salt, and garlic together in a blender
2. Add in lemon juice and mix
3. Add to the serving bowl and top with extra olive oil and cayenne pepper

Nutrition:
Carbs: 27.1g
Protein: 9.8g
Fats: 18.7g
Calories: 302Kcal

242. Simple Peas Mix

Preparation Time: 5minutes
Servings: 2

Ingredients

- Frozen peas: 1 cup can washed and drained
- Salt: as per your taste
- Pepper: as per your taste
- Cashew cream: ½ cup

Directions:
1. Combine all the ingredients
2. Serve as the side dish

Nutrition:
Carbs: 10g
Protein: 5g
Fats: 6.5g
Calories: 133Kcal

243. Spinach Green Hummus

Preparation Time: 10 minutes
Servings: 4 as a side dish

Ingredients

- Chickpeas: 2 cups drained and rinsed
- Spinach: 1 cup
- Pistachios: 1 cup finely shredded
- Tahini: 3 tbsp
- Garlic: 1 clove
- Lemon juice: 2 tbsp
- Salt: as per your need
- Sesame seed: ½ tsp
- Water: 3 tbsp

Directions:
1. Blend spinach, chickpeas, tahini, water, salt, and garlic together in a blender
2. Add in lemon juice and mix
3. Add to the serving bowl and top with sesame seeds and pistachios

Nutrition:

Carbs: 34.2g
Protein: 16.9g
Fats:22.7g
Calories: 295Kcal

244. Stir-Fry Greens

Preparation Time: 30 minutes
Servings: 2

Ingredients

- Long-stemmed broccoli: 1 cup
- Kale: 1 cup
- Olive oil: 1 tbsp
- Peas: 1 cup
- Salt: as per your taste
- Smoked paprika: ½ tsp

Directions:
1. Take a pan and heat olive oil
2. Take a bowl and add broccoli, peas, salt, paprika and mix well and add to the pan
3. Fry on low heat for 20 minutes and turn in between
4. Add kale at the last minutes
5. Serve as a salad with the main dish

Nutrition:
Carbs: 21.5g
Protein:9.4g
Fats: 9.55g
Calories: 127.2Kcal
Rice Milk

245. Preparation Time: 20 minutes plus overnight soaking

Servings: 400ml

Ingredients

- Rice: 250g
- Maple syrup: 2 tsp
- Water: 500 ml

Directions:
1. Toast rice in the pan lightly and soak overnight in 250ml water

2. Add maple syrup, rice, and 250ml water to the blender and blend till smoothen
3. Strain and discard the puree
4. Shake before serving

Nutrition:

Carbs: 7.5g

Protein: 0.4g

Fats: 0.1g

Calories: 33Kcal

246. Roasted Chili Potatoes

Preparation Time: 35 minutes

Servings: 2

Ingredients

- Olive oil: 1 tbsp
- Potatoes: 2 cups cut like fries
- Salt: as per your taste
- Pepper: as per your taste
- Red chili flakes: 1 tsp

Directions:

1. Preheat the oven 200C
2. Add potatoes to the baking sheet and sprinkle seasoning and brush with olive oil
3. Roast for 25 minutes till it turns golden and soft
4. Remove from the oven and sprinkle red chili flakes
5. Serve as the side dish

Nutrition:

Carbs: 26 g

Protein: 3g

Fats: 7.2g

Calories: 178Kcal

247. Roasted Parsnips With Zhoug

Preparation Time: 35 minutes

Servings: 4

Ingredients

- Parsnips: 4 thickly sliced
- Salt and pepper: as per your taste
- Olive oil: 1 tbsp

For the Zhoug:

- Flat-leaf parsley: ½ cup chopped
- Coriander: ½ cup chopped
- Vinegar: 1 tbsp
- Green chili: 1 chopped
- Garlic:½ clove chopped
- Ground cumin: ½ tsp

Directions:

1. Preheat the oven to 200C
2. Take a baking sheet and place parsnips
3. Brush oil and sprinkle salt and pepper
4. Bake for 25-30 minutes till they tender
5. In the meanwhile, add all the zhoug ingredients to the food processor and blend
6. Add 3-4 tablespoons of water if needed
7. Serve roasted parsnips with zhoug

Nutrition:

Carbs: 24g

Protein: 1.6g

Fats: 3.9g

Calories: 141Kcal

248. Roasted Broccoli With Peanuts And Kecap Manis

Preparation Time: 40 minutes

Servings: 4

Ingredients

- Broccoli: a large head diced
- Vegetable oil: 1 tbsp
- Kecap manis: 4 tbsp
- Spring onions: 2 sliced
- Grated garlic: 2 cloves
- Sesame oil: 2 tbsp

- Ginger: 1 tbsp grated
- Dried chili flakes: a pinch
- Salted peanuts: a handful roughly chopped
- Rice vinegar: 3 tbsp
- Coriander: ½ cup chopped
- Ready-made crispy onions: 3 tbsp
- Water: 50ml
- Cooked jasmine rice to serve

Directions:
1. Preheat the oven to 180C
2. Take a large pan and add oil and fry broccoli in batches and spread on baking sheet
3. In the same pan, fry garlic, ginger, and chili flakes for a minute and then add rice vinegar, manis, sesame oil, and water
4. Pour all of this mixture over broccoli and cover with foil
5. Roast the broccoli for 20 minutes in the oven
6. Mix crispy onion and salted peanuts together and sprinkle over cooked broccoli
7. Top with coriander and serve with rice

Nutrition:
Carbs: 22.5 g
Protein: 9.4 g
Fats: 12.8 g
Calories:258 Kcal

249. Roasted Red Cabbage Pesto

Preparation Time: 10 minutes
Servings: 4 as a side dish

Ingredients
- Red cabbage: 1 head small
- Garlic: 2 cloves
- Lemon juice: 3 tbsp
- Ground almonds: 2 tbsp
- Extra-virgin olive oil: 3 tbsp
- Salt: as per your need
- Chili sauce: 1 tbsp

Directions:
1. Roast cabbage in the oven for 10 minutes at 160C
2. Take a blender and add all the ingredients including roasted cabbage
3. Blend them well
4. Serve with crispy chips

Nutrition:
Carbs: 11.8g
Protein: 10.4g
Fats: 34.2g
Calories: 366Kcal

250. Roasted Garlic Toasts

Preparation Time: 45 minutes
Servings: 4

Ingredients
- Whole bulbs garlic: 4
- Olive oil: 400ml
- Cherry tomatoes: 300g halved
- Sprigs thyme: 6
- Toasted sourdough: 4 slices

Directions:
1. Preheat the oven to medium heat
2. Cut the garlic horizontally and sprinkle thyme and salt, and add to the bowl filled with oil
3. Place in the oven and Cooking Time: for 25 minutes till garlic becomes soft
4. Remove from the oven and spread on the toasted sourdough
5. Top with cherry tomatoes and serve

Nutrition:
Carbs: 38 g
Protein: 8.8 g
Fats: 18.2 g
Calories: 358 Kcal

251. Roasted Olive Oil Tomatoes

Preparation Time: 1 hour 50 minutes
Servings: 5

Ingredients

- Cherry tomatoes on the vine: 4-6 bunches
- Bay leaves: 6
- Olive oil: 200ml
- Garlic: 1 whole bulb cut in ½
- Crusty bread warmed to serve

Directions:

1. Heat the oven to 150C
2. Put the garlic and tomatoes in a baking dish, now add bay leaves and season
3. Pour the olive oil on a baking dish and cover it with foil
4. Let it bake for 1 ½ hour and then serve it with crusty bread

Nutrition:
Carbs: 4.6g
Protein: 1.3g
Fats: 33.6g
Calories: 328Kcal

252. Rocket Chickpeas Salad

Preparation Time: 15 minutes
Servings: 2

Ingredients

- Avocado: 1 cut into small pieces
- Chickpeas: 400g can drained and rinsed
- Red chili: 1 chopped
- Cumin seeds: 1 tsp
- Red onion: 1/2 finely chopped
- Roasted red peppers: 3 chopped
- Olive oil
- Lime: 1 plus wedges to serve
- Rocket: 2 handfuls
- Pitta bread: 2 warmed

Directions:

1. Mix onion, avocado, peppers, chickpeas, and chili in a bowl
2. Take two tablespoons of olive oil and whisk it with lime juice while adding seasoning and cumin seeds
3. Put it in the bowl and mix well
4. Add the chickpeas mixture to the rocket pile into 2 plates
5. Best served with warm pittas

Nutrition:
Carbs: 60.4g
Protein: 18.3g
Fats: 26.4g
Calories: 586Kcal

253. Savory Broccoli Mash

Preparation Time: 30 minutes
Servings: 4 as a side dish

Ingredients

- Broccoli: 2 cups florets
- Spinach: 1 cup
- Tahini: 2 tbsp
- Garlic: 1 clove
- Vinegar: 1 tbsp
- Pepper: as per your need
- Salt: as per your need

Directions:

1. Take a pan and boil salt and water
2. Add broccoli in the salted water and cover and Cooking Time: for 20 minutes and add spinach at the end
3. Drain and mash using a potato masher and add to the bowl
4. Mix tahini, olive oil, vinegar, salt, pepper, and garlic together
5. Add this dressing to the broccoli mixture and combine well

Nutrition:

Carbs: 5.5g
Protein: 4.07g
Fats: 14.5g
Calories: 178Kcal

254. Savory Mango Chat

Preparation Time: 5 minutes
Servings: 4

Ingredients

- Mango: 4 peeled and diced into bite-sized chunks
- Chaat masala: 2 tsp
- Lime: 1 juiced
- Sea salt: ½ tsp
- Coconut yogurt to serve

Directions:

1. Place all the ingredients in a large bowl and shake them well
2. Now serve it with some coconut yogurt if you desire

Nutrition:
Carbs:50 g
Protein:2.8 g
Fats:1.3 g
Calories: 201Kcal

255. Som Tam Salad

Preparation Time: 20 minutes and marinating as well
Servings: 2

Ingredients

- Green beans: 110g cooked and divided
- Courgettes: 2
- Cherry tomatoes: 120g halved
- Carrot: 1 shredded
- Lime: 1 juiced
- Palm sugar: 1 tbsp
- Tamari: 1 tbsp
- Coriander: ¼ cup chopped
- Mint: ¼ cup chopped
- Chili: 1 finely sliced
- Roasted peanuts: 1 tbsp chopped

Directions:

1. With the spiraliser, create thin strands of courgette
2. Add green beans, cherry tomatoes, carrots, lime juice, palm sugar, and chili and give pulse in the blender or crush in pestle and mortar
3. Add the mixture to the courgette and mix for 15 minutes
4. Top with chopped peanuts, mint, and coriander, combine well and serve

Nutrition:
Carbs: 20.6 g
Protein: 8.9 g
Fats: 5.2 g
Calories: 178 Kcal

SOUPS AND STEWS

256. Herby Cheddar Soup

Preparation Time: 12 minutes
Cooking Time: 23 minutes
Serving Size: 4
Ingredients:

- 5 tbsp butter
- 6 slices vegan bacon, chopped
- 1 small yellow onion, roughly chopped
- 3 garlic cloves, minced
- 2 tbsp finely chopped rosemary
- 1 tbsp chopped fresh oregano
- 1 tbsp chopped fresh tarragon
- 2 cups peeled and cubed parsnips
- 3 ½ cups vegetable broth
- Salt and freshly ground black pepper to taste
- 1 cup unsweetened almond milk
- 1 cup grated cheddar cheese
- 2 tbsp chopped scallions for garnishing

Directions:

1. Over medium heat, melt 1 tablespoon of butter in a large saucepan. Fry in vegan bacon until browned and crispy, 5 minutes. Transfer to a paper towel-lined plate and set aside.
2. Melt remaining butter in the same pot and sauté onion, garlic, rosemary, oregano, and tarragon until fragrant, 3 minutes.
3. Stir in parsnips and vegetable broth, season with salt and black pepper, and Cooking Time: (covereduntil parsnips soften, 10 to 12 minutes.
4. Using an immersion blender, process ingredients until smooth. Stir in almond milk and cheddar cheese;

simmer with frequent stirring until cheese melts, 3 minutes.
5. Divide soups into serving bowls, top with vegan bacon, and garnish with scallions.
6. Serve warm with low carb bread.

Nutrition:
Calories 775, Total Fat 57.42g, Total Carbs 8.63g, Fiber 2.1g, Net Carbs 6.53g, Protein 18.2g

257. Creamy Onion Soup

Preparation Time: 15 minutes
Cooking Time: 1 hour 5 minutes
Serving Size: 4
Ingredients:

- 1 tbsp olive oil
- 2 tbsp butter
- 3 cups thinly sliced white onions
- 2 garlic cloves, pressed
- ½ cup dry white wine
- 2 tsp almond flour
- 3 tbsp freshly chopped rosemary
- Salt and freshly ground black pepper to taste
- 2 cups hot vegetable broth
- 2 cups unsweetened almond milk
- 1 cup grated Pecorino Romano cheese

Directions:

1. Over medium fire, heat olive oil and butter in a large pot. Sauté onions until softened, 10 minutes, stirring regularly to avoid browning. Reduce heat to low and continue cooking for 15 minutes.
2. Add garlic; Cooking Time: further until onions caramelize while still stirring, 10 minutes.
3. Stir in white wine, almond flour, and increase heat. Season with rosemary, salt, and black pepper, and pour in

124

vegetable broth. Cover pot, allow boiling, and then simmer for 30 minutes.

4. Pour in almond milk and half of Pecorino Romano cheese. Stir until cheese melts; adjust taste with salt and black pepper.

5. Spoon soup into serving bowls, top with remaining cheese, and serve warm.

Nutrition:
Calories 340, Total Fat 23.43g, Total Carbs 7.24g, Fiber 1.6g, Net Carbs 5.64g, Protein 15.15g

258. Creamy Tofu Mushroom Soup

Preparation Time: 10 minutes
Cooking Time: 14 minutes
Serving Size: 4
Ingredients:

- 1 tbsp olive oil
- 2/3 cup sliced white button mushrooms
- 1 large white onion, finely chopped
- 1 garlic clove, minced
- 1 tsp ginger puree
- 1 cup vegetable broth
- 2 turnips, peeled and chopped
- Salt and freshly ground black pepper to taste
- 2 (14 ozsilken tofu, drained and rinsed
- 2 cups unsweetened almond milk
- 1 tbsp freshly chopped oregano
- 1 tbsp freshly chopped parsley to garnish
- 1 tbsp chopped walnuts for topping

Directions:
1. Over medium fire, heat olive oil in a large saucepan and Cooking Time: mushrooms until softened, 5 minutes.

Remove onto a plate and set aside.

2. Add and sauté onion, garlic, and ginger puree until fragrant and soft.

3. Pour in vegetable broth, turnips, salt, and black pepper. Cooking Time: until turnips soften, 6 minutes.

4. Add silken tofu and using an immersion blender, puree ingredients until very smooth.

5. Stir in mushrooms and simmer until mushrooms heat through, 2 to 3 minutes. Make sure to stir soup frequently to prevent tofu from curdling.

6. Add almond milk and adjust taste with salt and black pepper. Stir in oregano and dish soup.

7. Garnish with parsley and serve with soy chorizo chips.

Nutrition:
Calories 923, Total Fat 8.59g, Total Carbs 12.23g, Fiber 4.8g, Net Carbs 7.43g, Protein 23.48g

259. Kale-Ginger Soup With Poached Eggs

Preparation Time: 10 minutes
Cooking Time: 16 minutes
Serving Size: 4
Ingredients:

- 1 tbsp butter
- ½ tbsp sesame oil + extra for topping
- 1 small onion, finely sliced
- 3 garlic cloves, minced
- 2 tsp ginger paste
- 2 cups chopped baby kale
- 2 cups chopped green beans
- 3 tbsp freshly chopped parsley + extra for garnish
- 4 cups vegetable stock
- Salt and freshly ground black pepper

to taste
- 3 cups water
- 4 eggs

Directions:
1. Over medium heat, melt butter and sesame oil in a large pot. Sauté onion and garlic until softened and fragrant, 3 minutes. Stir in ginger and Cooking Time: for 2 minutes.
2. Add kale, allowing wilting, and pour in green beans, parsley, and vegetable stock. Season with salt and black pepper. Cover and allow boiling; reduce heat, and simmer for 7 to 10 minutes.
3. Meanwhile, bring water to simmer in a medium pot over medium heat. Swirl water with a spoon and poach eggs in water one after another, 4 minutes. Remove onto a paper towel-lined plate to drain water.
4. Turn soup's heat off and pour ingredients into a blender. Puree until very smooth and divide into four bowls.
5. Top each with an egg, sesame oil, and parsley.

Nutrition:
Calories 463, Total Fat 30.05g, Total Carbs 8.5g, Fiber 2.7g, Net Carbs 5.8g, Protein 23.69g

260. Broccoli And Collard Soup

Preparation Time: 15 minutes
Cooking Time: 18 minutes
Serving Size: 4
Ingredients:
- 1 tbsp olive oil
- 2 tbsp butter
- 1 medium brown onion, thinly sliced
- 3 garlic cloves, finely sliced
- 1 large head broccoli, cut into florets

- 4 cups vegetable stock
- 2 cups collards
- ¼ cup freshly chopped parsley
- Salt and freshly ground black pepper to taste
- 1 tbsp fresh dill leaves for garnishing
- 1 cup grated Parmesan cheese for topping

Directions:
1. Over medium fire, heat olive oil and butter in a large saucepan and sauté onion and garlic until softened and fragrant, 3 minutes.
2. Stir in broccoli and Cooking Time: until softened, 5 minutes.
3. Add vegetable stock, salt, and black pepper. Cover pot and allow boiling. Reduce heat and simmer until broccoli is very soft, 10 minutes.
4. Open lid and use an immersion blender to puree soup until completely smooth. Stir in collards, parsley, and adjust taste with salt and black pepper.
5. Dish soup, garnish with dill leaves and Parmesan cheese; serve warm.

Nutrition:
Calories 515, Total Fat 33.89g, Total Carbs 9.1g, Fiber 4.6g, Net Carbs 4.5g, Protein 38.33g

261. Chilled Lemongrass And Avocado Soup

Preparation Time: 5 minutes
Cooking Time: 5 minutes + 1 hour refrigeration
Serving Size: 4
Ingredients:
- 2 stalks lemongrass, chopped
- 2 cups chopped avocado pulp
- 2 cups vegetable broth
- 2 lemons, juiced

- 3 tbsp chopped mint leaves + extra to garnish
- Salt and freshly ground black pepper to taste
- 2 cups heavy cream

Directions:
1. In a large pot, add lemongrass, avocado, and vegetable broth; bring to a slow boil over low heat until lemongrass softens and avocado warms through, 5 minutes.
2. Stir in lemon juice, mint leaves, salt, black pepper, and puree ingredients with an immersion blender.
3. Stir in heavy cream and turn heat off.
4. Dish soup into serving bowls, chill for 1 hour, and garnish with some mint leaves. Serve.

Nutrition:
Calories 339, Total Fat 33.3g, Total Carbs 6.58g, Fiber 3g, Net Carbs 3.58g, Protein 3.59g

262. Turnip–Tomato Soup

Preparation Time: 15 minutes
Cooking Time: 33 minutes
Serving Size: 6
Ingredients:
- 1 tbsp butter
- 1 tbsp olive oil
- 1 large yellow onion, chopped
- 4 garlic cloves, minced
- 6 red bell peppers, deseeded and sliced
- 2 turnips, peeled and chopped
- 3 cups chopped tomatoes
- 4 cups vegetable stock
- Salt and freshly ground black pepper to taste
- 3 cups coconut milk
- 2 cups toasted chopped almonds
- 1 cup grated Parmesan cheese

Directions:
1. Over medium fire, heat butter and olive oil in a medium pot, and sauté onion and garlic until fragrant and soft, 3 minutes.
2. Stir in bell pepper and turnips; Cooking Time: until sweaty, 10 minutes.
3. Mix in tomatoes, vegetable stock, salt, and black pepper. Cover lid and Cooking Time: over low heat for 20 minutes.
4. Turn heat off and using an immersion blender, puree ingredients until smooth. Stir in coconut milk.
5. Pour soup into serving bowls and garnish with almonds and Parmesan cheese.
6. Serve immediately with low carb cheese bread.

Nutrition:
Calories 955, Total Fat 86.65g, Total Carbs 10.5g, Fiber 6.5g, Net Carbs 4g, Protein 19.11g

263. Spring Vegetable Soup

Preparation Time: 8 minutes
Cooking Time: 12 minutes
Serving Size: 4
Ingredients:
- 4 cups vegetable stock
- 3 cups green beans, chopped
- 2 cups asparagus, chopped
- 1 cup pearl onions, peeled and halved
- 2 cups seaweed mix (or spinach
- 1 tbsp garlic powder
- Salt and freshly ground white pepper to taste
- 2 cups grated Parmesan cheese, for serving

Directions:
1. In a large pot, add vegetable stock,

green beans, asparagus, and pearl onions. Season with garlic powder, salt and white pepper.

2. Cover pot and Cooking Time: over low heat until vegetables soften, 10 minutes.
3. Stir in seaweed mix and adjust taste with salt and white pepper.
4. Dish into serving bowls and top with plenty of Parmesan cheese.
5. Serve with low carb bread.

Nutrition:
Calories 196, Total Fat 11.9g, Total Carbs 10.02g, Fiber 5.7g, Net Carbs 4.32g

264. Zucchini-Dill Bowls With Ricotta Cheese

Preparation Time: 10 minutes
Cooking Time: 25 minutes
Serving Size: 4
Ingredients:

- 4 zucchinis, spiralized and chopped roughly
- Salt and freshly ground black pepper to taste
- ¼ tsp Dijon mustard
- 1 tbsp olive oil
- 1 tbsp freshly squeezed lemon juice
- ½ cup baby spinach
- 1 tbsp freshly chopped tarragon
- 2/3 cup ricotta cheese
- 2 tbsp toasted pine nuts

Directions:

1. Place zucchinis in a medium bowl and season with salt and black pepper.
2. In a small bowl, whisk mustard, olive oil, and lemon juice. Pour mixture over zucchini and toss well.
3. Add spinach, tarragon, ricotta cheese, and pine nuts. Mix with two ladles and serve.

Nutrition:
Calories 857, Total Fat 36.33g, Total Carbs 12.46g, Fiber 2.4g, Net Carbs 10.06g, Protein 26.13g

265. Cauliflower Soup

Preparation time: 10 minutes
Cooking time: 4 hours 5 minutes
Total time: 4 hours 15 minutes
Servings: 04
Ingredients:

- 2 tablespoons olive oil
- 1½ cups sweet white onion, chopped
- 2 large cloves of garlic, chopped
- 1 head cauliflower, cut into florets
- 1 cup coconut milk
- 1 cup filtered water
- 1 teaspoon vegetable stock paste
- 2 tablespoons nutritional yeast
- Dash of olive oil
- Fresh cracked pepper
- Parsley, to serve

How to prepare:

1. Add olive oil and onion to a slow cooker.
2. Sauté for 5 minutes then add the rest of the ingredients.
3. Put on the slow cooker's lid and Cooking Time: for 4 hours on low heat.
4. Once done, blend the soup with a hand blender.
5. Garnish with parsley, and cracked pepper
6. Serve.

Nutritional Values:
Calories 119
Total Fat 14 g
Saturated Fat 2 g
Cholesterol 65 mg
Sodium 269 mg

Total Carbs 19 g
Fiber 4 g
Sugar 6 g
Protein 5g

266. Greek Lentil Soup

Preparation time: 10 minutes
Cooking time: 6 hours 2 minutes
Total time: 6 hours 12 minutes
Servings: 04
Ingredients:

Soup:

- 1 cup lentils
- 1 medium sweet onion, chopped
- 2 large carrots, chopped
- 2 sticks of celery, chopped
- 4 cups veggie broth
- Olive oil to sauté
- 4 tablespoons tomato sauce
- 3 cloves garlic
- 3 bay leaves
- Salt, to taste
- Black pepper, to taste
- Dried oregano, to taste

Toppings:

- Vinegar
- Lemon juice
- Hot sauce

How to Prepare:
1. In a slow cooker, add olive oil and onion.
2. Sauté for 2 minutes then add the rest of the soup ingredients.
3. Put on the slow cooker's lid and Cooking Time: for 6 hours on low heat.
4. Serve warm with the vinegar, lemon juice, and hot sauce.

Nutritional Values:
Calories 231

Total Fat 20.1 g
Saturated Fat 2.4 g
Cholesterol 110 mg
Sodium 941 mg
Total Carbs 20.1 g
Fiber 0.9 g
Sugar 1.4 g
Protein 4.6 g

267. Broccoli White Bean Soup

Preparation time: 10 minutes
Cooking time: 4 hrs. 32 minutes
Total time: 4 hrs. 42 minutes
Servings: 04
Ingredients:

- 1 large bunch broccoli
- 3 cloves garlic
- 1 medium white potato
- ¼ cup carrot, chopped
- 2 cups almond milk
- 1½ cups white beans, cooked
- 1 white onion, chopped
- ¾ teaspoon black pepper
- ¼ teaspoon salt
- ½ teaspoon smoky paprika
- ⅓ cup nutritional yeast
- 1 bay leaf
- 1 cup cooked pasta

How to Prepare:
1. In a slow cooker, add olive oil and onion.
2. Sauté for 2 minutes then toss in the rest of the ingredients except pasta and beans.
3. Put on the slow cooker's lid and Cooking Time: for 4 hours on low heat.
4. Once done, add pasta and beans to the soup and mix gently.
5. Cover the soup and remove it from

the heat then leave it for another 30 minutes.

6. Serve warm.

Nutritional Values:

Calories 361

Total Fat 16.3 g

Saturated Fat 4.9 g

Cholesterol 114 mg

Sodium 515 mg

Total Carbs 29.3 g

Fiber 0.1 g

Sugar 18.2 g

Protein 3.3 g

268. African Lentil Soup

Preparation time: 10 minutes

Cooking time: 20 minutes

Total time: 30 minutes

Servings: 4

Ingredients:

- 1 teaspoon oil
- ½ medium onion, chopped
- 2 juicy tomatoes, chopped
- 4 garlic cloves, chopped
- 1-inch piece of ginger, chopped
- 1 tablespoon Sambal Oelek
- 1 tablespoon tomato paste
- 1½ teaspoons ground cumin
- 2 teaspoons ground coriander
- 1 teaspoon Harissa Spice Blend
- ¼ teaspoon black pepper
- ¼ cup nut butter
- 2 tablespoons peanuts
- ½ cup red lentils
- 2½ cups vegetable stock
- ¾ teaspoon salt
- 1 teaspoon lemon juice
- ½ cup packed baby spinach

How to Prepare:

1. In a slow cooker, add olive oil and onion.
2. Sauté for 5 minutes then toss in rest of the ingredients except peanuts.
3. Put on the slow cooker's lid and Cooking Time: for 5 hours on low heat.
4. Once done, garnish with peanuts.
5. Serve.

Nutritional Values:

Calories 205

Total Fat 22.7 g

Saturated Fat 6.1 g

Cholesterol 4 mg

Sodium 227 mg

Total Carbs 26.1 g

Fiber 1.4 g

Sugar 0.9 g

Protein 5.2 g

269. Artichoke Bean Soup

Preparation time: 10 minutes

Cooking time: 20 minutes

Total time: 30 minutes

Servings: 04

Ingredients:

- 1 (15 ouncecan artichoke hearts
- ½ bunch kale, chopped
- 2 cups vegetable broth
- 1 tablespoon dried basil
- 1 tablespoon dried oregano
- 1 teaspoon salt
- ½ teaspoon red pepper flakes
- Black pepper, to taste
- 2 (14 ouncecans roasted tomatoes, diced
- 1 (15 ouncecan white beans, drained

How to Prepare:

1. Add all ingredients to a saucepan.
2. Put on the saucepan's lid and Cooking

Time: for 20 minutes on a simmer.
3. Serve warm.

Nutritional Values:
Calories 201
Total Fat 8.9 g
Saturated Fat 4.5 g
Cholesterol 57 mg
Sodium 340 mg
Total Carbs 24.7 g
Fiber 1.2 g
Sugar 1.3 g
Protein 15.3 g

270. Chinese Rice Soup

Preparation time: 10 minutes
Cooking time: 3 hrs.
Total time: 3hrs. 10 minutes
Servings: 04
Ingredients:

Congee:

- 1 cup of white rice (uncooked
- 2-inch piece fresh ginger, minced
- 4 cloves garlic, minced
- 10 cups water
- 14 dried shiitake mushrooms

Toppings:

- Green onions
- Cilantro
- Sesame seeds
- Hot sauce
- Toasted sesame oil
- Soy sauce
- Peanuts
- Chili oil
- Shelled edamame

How to Prepare:
1. Add all the ingredients to a slow cooker.
2. Put on the slow cooker's lid and

Cooking Time: for 3 hours on low heat.
3. Once done, garnish with desired toppings.
4. Serve warm.

Nutritional Values:
Calories 210.6
Total Fat 10.91g
Saturated Fat 7.4g
Sodium 875 mg
Potassium 604 mg
Carbohydrates 25.6g
Fiber 4.3g
Sugar 7.9g
Protein 2.1g

271. Black-Eyed Pea Soup With Greens

Preparation time: 10 minutes
Cooking time: 5 hrs.
Total time: 5 hrs. 10 minutes
Servings: 04
Ingredients:

- ½ cup black eyed peas
- ½ cup brown lentils
- 1 teaspoon oil
- ½ teaspoon cumin seeds
- ½ cup onions, chopped
- 5 cloves garlic, chopped
- 1-inch piece of ginger chopped
- 1 teaspoon ground coriander
- ½ teaspoon ground cumin
- ½ teaspoon turmeric
- ¼ teaspoon black pepper
- ½ teaspoon cayenne powder
- 2 tomatoes, chopped
- ½ teaspoon lemon juice
- 1 teaspoon salt
- 2 ½ cups water
- ½ cup chopped spinach

- ½ cup small chopped green beans

How to Prepare:
1. Add olive oil and cumin seeds to a slow cooker.
2. Sauté for 1 minute then toss in the rest of the ingredients.
3. Put on the slow cooker's lid and Cooking Time: for 5 hours on low heat.
4. Once done, garnish as desired
5. Serve warm.

Nutritional Values:
Calories 197
Total Fat 4 g
Saturated Fat 0.5 g
Cholesterol 135 mg
Sodium 790 mg
Total Carbs 31 g
Fiber 12.2 g
Sugar 2.5 g
Protein 11 g

272. Beanless Garden Soup

Preparation time: 10 minutes
Cooking time: 4 hrs. 5 minutes
Total time: 4 hrs. 15 minutes
Servings: 04
Ingredients:

- 1 medium onion, diced
- 2 cloves garlic, minced
- 1 green bell pepper, diced
- 1 red bell pepper, diced
- 2 carrots, peeled and diced
- 1 medium zucchini, diced
- 1 small eggplant, diced
- 1 hot banana pepper, seeded and minced
- 1 jalapeño pepper, seeded and minced
- 1 can (28 ounce diced tomatoes
- 3 cups vegetable broth

- 1½ tablespoon chili powder
- 2 teaspoons smoked paprika
- 1 tablespoon cumin
- 2 tablespoons fresh oregano, chopped
- 2 tablespoons fresh cilantro, chopped
- Salt and black pepper to taste
- A few dashes of liquid smoke

How to Prepare:
1. In a slow cooker, add olive oil and onion.
2. Sauté for 5 minutes then toss in the rest of the ingredients.
3. Put on the slow cooker's lid and Cooking Time: for 4 hours on low heat.
4. Once done mix well.
5. Serve warm.

Nutritional Values:
Calories 305
Total Fat 11.8 g
Saturated Fat 2.2 g
Cholesterol 56 mg
Sodium 321 mg
Total Carbs 34.6 g
Fibers 0.4 g
Sugar 2 g
Protein 7 g

273. Black-Eyed Pea Soup With Olive Pesto

Preparation time: 10 minutes
Cooking time: 3 hrs. 5 minutes
Total time: 3 hrs. 15 minutes
Servings: 04
Ingredients:
Soup:

- 1 leek, trimmed
- 1 tablespoon olive oil
- 1 clove garlic, chopped
- 1 small carrot, chopped

- 1 stem fresh thyme, chopped
- 1 (15 ouncecan black-eyed peas, drained and rinsed
- 2½ cups vegetable broth
- ½ teaspoon salt
- ¼ teaspoon black pepper

Pesto:

- 1¼ cups pitted green olives
- ¼ cup parsley leaves
- 1 clove garlic
- 1 teaspoon capers, drained
- 1 tablespoon olive oil

How to Prepare:

1. In a slow cooker, add olive oil, carrot, leek, and garlic.
2. Sauté for 5 minutes then toss in the rest of the soup ingredients.
3. Put on the slow cooker's lid and Cooking Time: for 3 hours on low heat.
4. Meanwhile, blend the pesto ingredients in a blender until smooth.
5. Blend the soup in the slow cooker with a hand mixer.
6. Top with prepared pesto.
7. Serve warm.

Nutritional Values:

Calories 72
Total Fat 15.4 g
Saturated Fat 4.2 g
Cholesterol 168 mg
Sodium 203 mg
Total Carbs 28.5 g
Sugar 1.1 g
Fiber 4 g
Protein 7.9 g

274. Spinach Soup With Basil

Preparation time: 10 minutes
Cooking time: 5hrs. 5 minutes
Total time: 5 hrs. 15 minutes
Servings: 06
Ingredients:

- 8 ounces potatoes, diced
- 1 medium onion, chopped
- 1 large clove of garlic, chopped
- 1 teaspoon powdered mustard
- 3 cups water
- ¼ teaspoon salt
- Ground cayenne pepper
- ½ cup packed fresh dill
- 10 ounces frozen spinach

How to Prepare:

1. In a low cooker, add olive oil and onion.
2. Sauté for 5 minutes then toss in rest of the soup ingredients.
3. Put on the slow cooker's lid and Cooking Time: for 5 hours on low heat.
4. Once done, puree the soup with a hand blender.
5. Serve warm.

Nutritional Values:

Calories 162
Total Fat 4 g
Saturated Fat 1.9 g
Cholesterol 25 mg
Sodium 101 mg
Total Carbs 17.8 g
Sugar 2.1 g
Fiber 6 g
Protein 4 g

275. Red Lentil Salsa Soup

Preparation time: 10 minutes
Cooking time: 17 minutes
Total time: 27 minutes
Servings: 06
Ingredients:

- 1¼ cups red lentils, rinsed
- 4 cups of water
- ½ cup diced red bell pepper
- 1¼ cups red salsa
- 1 tablespoon chili powder
- 1 tablespoon dried oregano
- 1 teaspoon smoked paprika
- ¼ teaspoon black pepper
- ¾ cup frozen sweet corn
- Salt to taste
- 2 tablespoons lime juice

How to Prepare:

1. In a saucepan, add all the ingredients except the corn.
2. Put on saucepan's lid and Cooking Time: for 15 minutes at a simmer.
3. Stir in corn and Cooking Time: for another 2 minutes.
4. Serve.

Nutritional Values:
Calories 119
Total Fat 14 g
Saturated Fat 2 g
Cholesterol 65 mg
Sodium 269 mg
Total Carbs 19 g
Fiber 4 g
Sugar 6 g
Protein 5g

276. Caldo Verde A La Mushrooms

Preparation time: 10 minutes
Cooking time: 5 hrs. 5 minutes
Total time: 5 hrs. 15 minutes
Servings: 08
Ingredients:

- ¼ cup olive oil
- 10 ounces button mushrooms, cleaned, and sliced
- 1½ teaspoons smoked paprika
- 1 pinch ground cayenne pepper
- 1 teaspoon salt
- 1 large onion, diced
- 2 cloves garlic, minced
- 2 pounds russet potatoes, peeled and diced
- 7 cups vegetable broth
- 8 ounces kale, sliced
- ½ teaspoon black pepper

How to Prepare:

1. In a pan, heat cooking oil and sauté mushrooms for 12 minutes.
2. Season the mushrooms with salt, cayenne pepper, and paprika.
3. Add olive oil and onion to a slow cooker.
4. Sauté for 5 minutes then toss in rest of the soup ingredients.
5. Put on the slow cooker's lid and Cooking Time: for 5 hours on low heat.
6. Once done, puree the soup with a hand blender.
7. Stir in sautéed mushrooms.
8. Serve.

Nutritional Values:
Calories 231
Total Fat 20.1 g
Saturated Fat 2.4 g
Cholesterol 110 mg
Sodium 941 mg
Total Carbs 20.1 g
Fiber 0.9 g

Sugar 1.4 g
Protein 4.6 g

277. Shiitake Mushroom Split Pea Soup

Preparation time: 10 minutes
Cooking time: 6 hours
Total time: 6 hours 10 minutes
Servings: 12
Ingredients:

- 1 cup dried, green split peas
- 2 cups celery, chopped
- 2 cups sliced carrots
- 1½ cups cauliflower, chopped
- 2 ounces dried shiitake mushrooms, chopped
- 9 ounces frozen artichoke hearts
- 11 cups water
- 1 teaspoon garlic powder
- 1½ teaspoon onion powder
- ½ teaspoon black pepper
- 1 tablespoon parsley
- ½ teaspoon ginger
- ½ teaspoon ground mustard seed
- ½ tablespoon brown rice vinegar

How to Prepare:
1. Add all the ingredients to a slow cooker.
2. Put on the slow cooker's lid and Cooking Time: for 6 hours on low heat.
3. Once done, garnish as desired.
4. Serve warm.

Nutritional Values:
Calories 361
Total Fat 16.3 g
Saturated Fat 4.9 g
Cholesterol 114 mg
Sodium 515 mg
Total Carbs 29.3 g

Fiber 0.1 g
Sugar 18.2 g
Protein 3.3 g

278. Velvety Vegetable Soup

Preparation time: 10 minutes
Cooking time: 2hrs 2 minutes
Total time: 2 hrs. 12 minutes
Servings: 4
Ingredients:

- ½ sweet onion, chopped
- 4 garlic cloves, chopped
- 1 small head broccoli, chopped
- 2 stalks celery, chopped
- 1 cup green peas
- 3 green onions, chopped
- 2¾ cups vegetable broth
- 4 cups leafy greens
- 1 (15 ouncecan of cannellini beans
- Juice from 1 lemon
- 2 tablespoons fresh dill, chopped
- 5 fresh mint leaves
- 1 teaspoon salt
- ½ cup coconut milk
- Fresh herbs and peas, to garnish

How to Prepare:
1. In a slow cooker, add olive oil and onion.
2. Sauté for 2 minutes then toss in the rest of the soup ingredients.
3. Put on the slow cooker's lid and Cooking Time: for 2 hours on low heat.
4. Once done, blend the soup with a hand blender.
5. Garnish with fresh herbs and peas.
6. Serve warm.

Nutritional Values:
Calories 205
Total Fat 22.7 g

Saturated Fat 6.1 g
Cholesterol 4 mg
Sodium 227 mg
Total Carbs 26.1 g
Fiber 1.4 g
Sugar 0.9 g
Protein 5.2 g

279. Sweet Potato And Peanut Soup

Preparation time: 10 minutes
Cooking time: 4 hrs. 5 minutes
Total time: 4 hrs. 15 minutes
Servings: 06
Ingredients:

- 1 tablespoon water
- 6 cups sweet potatoes, peeled and chopped
- 2 cups onions, chopped
- 1 cup celery, chopped
- 4 large cloves garlic, chopped
- 1 teaspoon salt
- 2 teaspoons cumin seeds
- 3½ teaspoons ground coriander
- 1 teaspoon paprika
- ½ teaspoon crushed red pepper flakes
- 2 cups vegetable stock
- 3 cups water
- 4 tablespoons fresh ginger, grated
- 2 tablespoons natural peanut butter
- 2 cups cooked chickpeas
- 4 tablespoons lime juice
- Fresh cilantro, chopped
- Chopped peanuts, to garnish

How to Prepare:

1. In a slow cooker, add olive oil and onion.
2. Sauté for 5 minutes then toss in the rest of the soup ingredients except chickpeas.
3. Put on the slow cooker's lid and Cooking Time: for 4 hours on low heat.
4. Once done, blend the soup with a hand blender.
5. Stir in chickpeas and garnish with cilantro and peanuts.
6. Serve warm.

Nutritional Values:
Calories 201
Total Fat 8.9 g
Saturated Fat 4.5 g
Cholesterol 57 mg
Sodium 340 mg
Total Carbs 24.7 g
Fiber 1.2 g
Sugar 1.3 g
Protein 15.3 g

280. 3-Ingredient Carrot And Red Lentil Soup

Preparation Time: 40 minutes
Servings: 3

Ingredients

- Split red lentils: 1 cup
- Carrots: 1 cup grated
- Water: 6 cups
- Onion: 1 large coarsely chopped
- Fine sea salt: as per your taste

Directions:

1. Take a large saucepan and add water and bring to boil
2. Add the chopped onions, carrots, lentils and salt and bring to boil
3. Lower the heat to medium and Cooking Time: for 20 minutes with partial cover
4. Add the mixture to the high-speed blender to make a puree
5. Whisk in water if desired

6. Add again to the pan and slowly heat on a low flame for 10-15 minutes
7. Add herbs or spices in between to augment the taste

Nutrition:

Carbs: 15.3 g

Protein: 6.2 g

Fats: 0.3 g

Calories: 90 Kcal

281. 3-Ingredient Enchilada Soup

Preparation Time: 25 minutes

Servings: 3

Ingredients

- Tomatoes: 1 cup crushed
- Vegan red enchilada sauce: 1.5 cups
- Black beans: 2 cups can rinsed and drained

Directions:

1. Take a medium-sized saucepan and add crushed tomatoes and enchilada sauce
2. Heat on a medium flame to thicken it for 6-8 minutes
3. Add beans to the pan and lower the heat to a minimum
4. Cooking Time: for 8-10 minutes
5. Serve with any toppings if you like

Nutrition:

Carbs: 27.4 g

Protein: 11g

Fats: 1 g

Calories: 166.4 Kcal

282. 3- Ingredient Lentil Soup

Preparation Time: 50 minutes

Servings: 2

Ingredients

- Brown lentils: 1 ¼ cups
- Fresh rosemary leaves: 2 ½ tbsp

minced
- Onion: 1 large chopped
- Sea salt: as per your taste
- Black pepper: ¼ tsp
- Water: 6 cups

Directions:

1. Take a large saucepan and add 1/3 cup of water and bring to boil
2. Add the chopped onions and lower the heat to medium
3. Stir with intervals for 10 minutes till onion changes color
4. Add salt, pepper, and rosemary and continue to stir for a minutes
5. Add lentils and remaining water to the pan and cover and Cooking Time: for 20 minutes
6. Lower the heat and continue simmering for 15 more minutes
7. Stir and break some lentils in the final minutes
8. Blend the soup if you like a creamy texture
9. Add more salt and pepper if needed and serve

Nutrition:

Carbs: 20 g

Protein: 8.5 g

Fats: 0.4 g

Calories: 150 Kcal

283. All Spices Lentils Bean Soup

Preparation Time: 45 minutes

Servings: 4

Ingredients

- Red lentils: 1 cup washed and drained
- Carrot: 2 medium chopped
- Beans: 1 cup drained
- Water: 3 cups
- Garlic: 3 cloves minced

- Onion: 1 medium finely chopped
- Ground cumin: 1 tsp
- Nutmeg: 1 tsp
- Ground coriander: 1 tsp
- Ground allspice: 1 tsp
- Ground cinnamon: 1 tsp
- Ground cayenne: ½ tsp
- Black pepper: as per your taste
- Extra virgin olive oil: 2 tbsp
- Salt: as per your taste
- Cilantro: 1 tbsp chopped

Directions:
1. Take a soup pot and heat oil in it on a medium flame
2. Add onion and fry for 4-5 minutes
3. Add carrot and garlic and stir for 5 minutes
4. Wash lentils and add them to the pot
5. Add water and bring to boil
6. Lower the heat and Cooking Time: and cover for 15 minutes till lentil softens
7. Add the remaining ingredients except for cilantro and Cooking Time: for an additional 15 minutes
8. Serve warm with cilantro on top

Nutrition:
Carbs: 425 g
Protein: 8.17 g
Fats: 4 g
Calories: 148.75 Kcal

284. Asparagus Cashew Cream Soup

Preparation Time: 30 minutes
Servings: 2

Ingredients
- Asparagus: 2 cups
- Vegetable stock: 4 cups
- Sesame seed: 2 tbsp
- Lemon juice: 1 tbsp
- Garlic: 4 cloves crushed
- Cashew cream: ½ cup
- Onion: 1 chopped
- Olive oil: 2 tbsp
- Salt & pepper: as per your taste

Preparation
1. Take a large saucepan and add olive oil to it
2. Fry onion and garlic till it turns golden brown
3. Chop asparagus and add to the pan along with the vegetable stock
4. Let it boil and then Cooking Time: on low heat for 20 minutes
5. When ready, add sesame seeds, lemon juice, and salt and pepper as per your taste
6. Serve with cashew cream on top

Nutrition:
Carbs: 11 g
Protein: 9.4 g
Fats: 18.3 g
Calories: 243.5 Kcal

285. Artichoke Spinach Soup

Preparation Time: 20 minutes
Servings: 3

Ingredients
- Cannellini beans: 1 cup rinsed and drained
- Artichoke hearts: 2 cups drained and chopped
- Frozen chopped spinach: 2 cups
- Water: 3 cups + 1 cup
- Garlic: 4 cloves chopped
- Onion: 1 medium chopped
- Italian herb blend: 2 tsp
- Sea salt: as per your taste
- Black pepper: as per your taste

Directions:

1. Take a blender and add onion, garlic, drained beans, salt, herb blend, and pepper and add water
2. Blend to give a smooth texture
3. Add this puree to a large pan and Cooking Time: on medium-high heat
4. When it initiates to boil, lower the heat and stir in between
5. Let the mixture to thicken a bit
6. Add one cup of water and spinach and blend
7. Also, add artichokes and heat for 5 minutes
8. Season with salt and pepper if desired and serve

Nutrition:
Carbs: 29.86 g
Protein: 12.9 g
Fats: 1.2 g
Calories: 144 Kcal

286. Beans With Garam Masala Broth

Preparation Time: 40 minutes
Servings: 2

Ingredients

- Red lentils: 1 cups
- Tomatoes: 1 cup can diced
- Beans: 1 cup can rinsed and drained
- Garam masala: 1 tbsp
- Vegetable oil: 2 tbsp
- Onion: 1 cup chopped
- Garlic: 3 cloves minced
- Ground cumin: 2 tbsp
- Smoked paprika: 1 tsp
- Celery: 1 cup chopped
- Sea salt: 1 tsp
- Lime juice and zest: 3 tbsp
- Fresh cilantro: 3 tbsp chopped

- Water: 2 cups

Directions:

1. Take a large pot and add oil to it
2. On the medium flame, add garlic, celery and onion
3. Add salt, garam masala, and cumin to them and stir for 5 minutes till they turn brown
4. Add water, lentils, and tomatoes with the juice and bring to boil
5. Bring to boil and heat for 25-30 minutes on low flame
6. Add in lime juice and zest and beans of your choice and stir
7. Serve with cilantro on top

Nutrition:
Carbs: 51.5 g
Protein: 19.1 g
Fats: 15.3 g
Calories: 420 Kcal

287. Black Beans And Potato Soup

Preparation Time: 50 minutes
Servings: 4

Ingredients

- Potatoes: 2 cups peeled and diced
- Black beans can: 2 cups rinsed and drained
- Kale: 1 cup chopped
- Onion: 1 medium finely chopped
- Garlic: 4 cloves minced
- Olive oil: 2 tsp
- Fresh rosemary leaves: 2 tbsp minced
- Vegetable broth: 4 cups
- Salt and ground black pepper: as per your taste

Directions:

1. Take a large saucepan and add oil
2. On a medium heat, add onions and Cooking Time: for 6-8 minutes

3. A dd rosemary and garlic and stir for a minute
4. Add potatoes with salt and pepper and sauté for two minutes
5. Pour vegetable broth and bring to boil
6. Lower the heat and Cooking Time: for 30 minutes till potatoes become soft
7. By using the back of spoon mash a few potatoes
8. Add kale and beans to the soup and again Cooking Time: for 5 minutes till they tender
9. Remove the soup from heat and season with salt and pepper

Nutrition:
Carbs: 45.25 g
Protein: 10.4 g
Fats: 8.7 g
Calories: 264 Kcal

288. Black Bean Cashew Soup

Preparation Time: 35 minutes
Servings: 3

Ingredients

- Black beans: 1 cup can
- Cashew nuts: ½ cup
- Spinach: 2 cups chopped
- Onion: 1 medium
- Freshly grated ginger: 2 tbsp
- Curry powder: 1 tbsp mild
- Vegetable broth: 2 cups
- Olive oil: 2 tbsp
- Lemon juice: as per your taste
- Garlic: 3 cloves
- Salt: as per your taste
- Fresh coriander: 2 tbsp

Directions:
1. Take a large pan and add olive oil
2. Add onion and garlic and fry for a minute and add curry powder and ginger
3. Continue frying for 5 minutes to make onion soft
4. Add spinach and vegetable broth and Cooking Time: on a medium flame for 10 minutes
5. Now blend with the hand blender
6. Add sliced cashews and black beans
7. Add water if needed and simmer for 5 minutes
8. Serve with lemon juice and fresh coriander on top

Nutrition:
Carbs: 44.5g
Protein:21.7g
Fats: 20.26g
Calories: 312.66Kcal

289. Black Beans Veggie Soup

Preparation Time: 45 minutes
Servings: 4

Ingredients

- Potatoes: 3 cups chopped
- Black beans: 1 cup can rinsed and drained
- Celery: 4 stalks sliced
- Fresh rosemary: 3 sprigs
- Carrots: 4 large sliced
- Vegetable oil: 2 tbsp
- Garlic: 2 cloves minced
- Shallots: 2 small diced
- Vegetable broth: 4 cups
- Broccoli: 1 cup florets
- Kale: 1 cup chopped
- Salt and black pepper: as per your need

Directions:
1. Take a large pot and add oil to it
2. On the medium flame, add shallots, garlic, celery and onion

3. Add salt and pepper to them and stir for 5 minutes till they turn brown
4. Now add potatoes and broccoli and again season with salt and pepper and sauté for two minutes
5. Pour vegetable broth and add rosemary and bring the mixture to boil
6. Lower the heat now and let it Cooking Time: for 20 minutes till potatoes soften
7. Include kale and black beans; stir, cover, and Cooking Time: for 5 minutes
8. Adjust the overall seasoning and add salt and pepper if needed

Nutrition:
Carbs: 43.5g
Protein: 7.72g
Fats: 8.6g
Calories: 248.5 Kcal

290. Broccoli Corn Soup

Preparation Time: 40 minutes
Servings: 2

Ingredients

- Corns: 2 cups can
- Broccoli: 1 cup
- Potato: 1 cup
- Spinach: 3 cups
- Garlic: 4 cloves
- Ginger root: 1 tbsp grated
- Spring onion: 4
- Turmeric: 1 tsp
- Lemon juice: 2 tbsp
- Coriander: ¼ cup chopped
- Ground coriander: 1 tsp
- Ground cumin: 1 tsp
- Salt and pepper: as per your taste
- Olive oil: 2 tbsp
- Vegetable broth: 4 cups

Directions:
1. In a large saucepan and heat olive oil
2. Crush garlic and chop white part of the green onion and sauté for a minute
3. Add coriander, cumin, ginger and turmeric and fry for a minute
4. Peel and dice potatoes, wash spinach, and separate broccoli florets and add to the pan
5. Sauté them for 5 minutes and add vegetable broth
6. Boil, and heat on low flame for 20 minutes
7. Blend the soup well and season with salt and pepper
8. Top with corns, lemon juice, and coriander leaves

Nutrition:
Carbs: 24.35g
Protein: 4.7g
Fats: 7.95g
Calories: 167.5Kcal

291. Brown Lentils Tomato Soup

Preparation Time: 40 minutes
Servings: 2

Ingredients

- Brown lentils: 1 cup
- Crushed tomatoes: 2 cups
- Onion: 1 diced
- Ginger: 1 tbsp paste
- Garlic: 1 tbsp paste
- Vegetable oil: 2 tbsp
- Water: 4 cups
- Italian herb seasoning: 1 tbsp
- Salt & pepper: as per your taste

Directions:
1. Take a large saucepan and add oil on a medium flame

2. Add onion and ginger and garlic paste and sauté for 3-4 minutes
3. Pour water and bring to boil
4. Add lentils and salt and bring to boil
5. Lower the heat to medium and Cooking Time: for 20 minutes with partial cover
6. Now add crushed tomatoes to the lentils along with herb seasoning and pepper
7. Cooking Time: on low flame for 15 minutes
8. Add the mixture to the high speed blender to make puree
9. Add salt and pepper to augment taste

Nutrition:
Carbs: 30.8g
Protein: 12.7g
Fats: 15.2g
Calories: 323.2Kcal

292. Brown Lentils Green Veggies Combo Soup

Preparation Time: 1 hour
Servings: 4-6

Ingredients

- Brown lentils: 150g
- Chickpeas: 400g can drained and rinsed
- Onion: 1 large finely chopped
- Leek: 2 diced
- Parsnips: 2 large finely diced
- Kale: 85g leaves shredded
- Olive oil: 2 tbsp
- Garlic: 2 cloves crushed
- Cayenne pepper: 1 tsp
- Coriander: a small bunch finely sliced
- Ground cinnamon: 1 tsp
- Ground turmeric: 1 tsp
- Ground coriander: 2 tsp

- Vegetable stock: 1 liter
- Lemons juice: 2 tbsp
- Salt: as per your need

Directions:
1. Take a large pan and heat olive oil in it
2. Add onions and parsnips and Cooking Time: them for 10 minutes
3. Then add coriander stalks and garlic and Cooking Time: for a minute and mix well
4. Next add spices and stir in lentils
5. Pour the stock and boil and then cover and Cooking Time: for 20 minutes and add leek at 10 minutes
6. Remove the lid and add in kale and chickpeas and stir
7. Sprinkle salt and pour in lemon juice
8. Top with coriander and serve

Nutrition:
Carbs: 29.4 g
Protein: 12.8 g
Fats: 7.2 g
Calories: 258 Kcal

293. Cannellini Beans Tomato Soup

Preparation Time: 30 minutes
Servings: 2

Ingredients

- Cannellini beans: 1 cup can
- Tomatoes: 1 cup chunks
- Tomatoes: 1 cup can
- Tomato paste: 2 tbsp
- Oregano: 2 tbsp dried
- Onion: 1 (finely chopped
- Garlic: 3 cloves (crushed
- Fresh basil: 1 small bunch
- Vegetable broth: 4 cups
- Salt & pepper: as per your taste
- Olive oil: 2 tbsp

Directions:

1. Take a large saucepan, heat olive oil in it
2. Add onion and garlic in it
3. Include tomato chunks, can chopped tomatoes, and tomato paste and combine them all together
4. Now add vegetable broth, oregano and fresh basil
5. Bring the mixture to boil and then lower the heat to medium and Cooking Time: for 15 minutes
6. Use the hand blender to blend the soup content and season with salt and pepper
7. Rinse, dry, and roast the cannellini beans
8. Add these beans on top of the soup and serve hot

Nutrition:
Carbs: 40g
Protein: 13.87g
Fats: 18.05g
Calories: 385.7Kcal

294. Cashew Chickpeas Soup

Preparation Time: 25 minutes
Servings: 2

Ingredients

- Chickpeas: 1 cup can
- Cashew nuts: ½ cup
- Spinach: 2 cups chopped
- Onion: 1 medium
- Freshly grated ginger: 2 tbsp
- Curry powder: 1 tbsp mild
- Vegetable broth: 2 cups
- Olive oil: 2 tbsp
- Lemon juice: as per your taste
- Garlic: 3 cloves
- Salt: as per your taste
- Fresh coriander: 2 tbsp

Directions:

1. Take a large pan and add olive oil
2. Add onion and garlic and fry for a minute and add curry powder and ginger
3. Continue frying for 5 minutes to make onion soft
4. Add spinach and vegetable broth and Cooking Time: on a medium flame for 10 minutes
5. Now blend with the hand blender and add sliced cashews and chickpeas
6. Add water if needed and simmer for 5 minutes
7. Serve with lemon juice and fresh coriander on top

Nutrition:
Carbs: 24.03g
Protein: 12.16g
Fats: 21.26g
Calories: 309 Kcal

SOUPS, STEWS & CHILIES

295. Cheesy Broccoli And Potato Soup

Preparation Time: 40 Minutes
Servings: 2
Ingredients:

- 2½ lb of potatoes, peeled and then chopped
- 3 carrots, chopped
- 1 broccoli head, chopped
- 4 cups water
- 2 tsp chili powder
- 1 tsp garlic powder
- ½ tsp smoked paprika
- 1 tsp turmeric
- 2 tsp salt
- 1/3 cup nutritional yeast
- ½ lemon, squeezed

Directions:

1. Place broccoli head on a trivet in iPot along with 1 cup water. Cover the pot with lid, switch on manual button and set the timer for 3 minutes. Once done, immediately release the steam. Remove broccoli, chop into small pieces.
2. Clean inner pot. Add potatoes to Instant Pot. Add carrots and remaining ingredients except for lemon juice and nutritional yeast.
3. Switch on manual button for 10 minutes over high pressure. Set steam release handle to 'sealing'. Once timer beeps, allow pressure to release naturally for 10 minutes and set handle to 'venting' to release any remaining steam.
4. Using an immersion blender, blend the soup until smooth. Add lemon juice and nutritional yeast and blend it again quickly.
5. Add in chopped broccoli now and just mix with a spoon and serve this!

296. Split Peas & Carrot Soup

Preparation Time: 35 Minutes
Servings: 3
Ingredients:

- 2 cups of green split peas
- 3-4 medium-sized carrots, chopped
- 1/2 of a large yellow onion, chopped
- 2 garlic cloves, minced
- 1/2 tsp of ground black pepper
- 4 cups of water
- 1 tbsp of veggie base or 1 bouillon cube (or 3 cups water with 3 cups veggie broth

Directions:

1. Add onion and garlic to Instant Pot along with 1/3 cup water and Switch the sautée button. Allow it to sautée for about 5 minutes till onions turn translucent.
2. Combine rest of the ingredients (except pepperin Instant Pot. Cover the pot with lid and switch manual button to 7 minutes over high pressure. Set steam release handle to 'sealing'.
3. When time is up, allow pressure to release naturally for 15 minutes. Let the soup cool down for some time. Add black pepper and using an immersion blender blend the soup so that still some chunks are left.
4. Add an additional ½ cup of water, if the soup is too thick.
5. Serve hot and enjoy.

297. Black Beans Soup

This black bean soup can be used as a delicious topping over steamed potatoes or rice.

Preparation Time: 70 Minutes
Servings: 2
Ingredients:

- 3 cups dry black beans, rinsed
- 1 carrot, chopped
- 1 yellow onion, diced
- 3 celery stalks, minced
- 4½ cups water
- 2 tsp vegetable base (or use 2 cups water with 2 cups veggie broth
- 6 garlic cloves, minced
- 1 tbsp cumin
- 1 tsp cayenne pepper
- 1 tsp chili powder
- Juice of 1 lime
- ¼ cup cilantro

Directions:

1. Rinse and drain beans.
2. Except for cilantro and lime juice, add all ingredients to Instant Pot and stir well. Set the vent on top to 'sealing' and cover with lid. Switch on manual button for 30 minutes over high pressure.
3. Once done, allow the steam to release naturally for about 15-20 minutes. Set the steam release handle to 'venting'.
4. Add cilantro and lime juice. use an immersion blender to lightly blend the soup.
5. Optionally some avocado, salsa or tortilla chips can be added to accompany this great soup!

298. Lentil And Mixed Vegetable Soup

Preparation Time: 40 Minutes
Servings: 3
Ingredients:

- 1 cup green lentils
- 5 potatoes, chopped
- 2 celery ribs, chopped
- 2 carrots, chopped
- 1 yellow onion, chopped
- 2 bay leaves
- 1 can (14.5 fl ozof diced tomatoes
- 1 cup green peas (frozen or canned
- 1 cup kale or spinach, finely chopped (fresh or frozen
- 3½ cups water
- 2 tsp black pepper
- 3 garlic cloves, minced
- 2 tsp vegetable base (or use 2 cups water with 2 cups veggie broth

Directions:

1. Chop potatoes, celery, carrots, onion and mince garlic and add them to Instant Pot along with rest of ingredients except for green peas and kale or spinach.
2. Cover with lid and set iPot manual for 10 minutes over high pressure. Once done allow steam to release naturally for about 15 minutes. Then release remaining steam using steam release handle. Open the lid.
3. Add green peas and kale or spinach. Stir the whole thing well. Let Instant Pot stay in 'Keep Warm' setting for around 10 minutes.
4. Remove bay leaves and serve the soup. When serving, add some salt or pepper to taste.

299. Pumpkin Stew

Preparation Time: 45 Minutes
Servings: 4
Ingredients:

- 21 oz sweet pumpkin, chopped
- 2 medium-sized onions, peeled and finely chopped
- 1 garlic clove
- 1 red pepper, finely chopped
- 1 tbsp of fresh tomato sauce
- ½ tbsp of chili powder
- 2 bay leaves
- 2 cups of red wine
- 1 cup of water
- 1 tsp of thyme, dry
- Salt and pepper to taste
- Oil for frying

Directions:

1. Plug in your instant pot and press "Sautee" button. Add chopped onions and stir-fry for 2 minutes. Add finely chopped red pepper, tomato sauce, and chili powder.
2. Continue to Cooking Time: until the pepper has softened.
3. Add the remaining ingredients and securely lock the lid. Adjust the steam release handle and set the timer for 8 minutes. Cooking Time: on high pressure.
4. When done, press "Cancel" button and release the steam naturally.
5. Enjoy!

300. Bean Onion Stew

Preparation Time: 30 Minutes
Servings: 6
Ingredients:

- 1 pound of fresh beans
- 1 large onion, chopped
- 4 cloves of garlic, finely chopped
- 3 ½ oz of olives, pitted
- 1 tbsp of ginger powder
- 1 tbsp of turmeric
- 1 tbsp of salt
- 4 cups of water

Directions:

1. Plug in your instant pot and press "Sautee" button. Heat up the oil and add onions and garlic. Stir-fry for 5 minutes, or until onions translucent.
2. Now, add the remaining ingredients and close the lid. Press "Manual" button and set the timer for 15 minutes. Adjust the steam release and Cooking Time: on high pressure.
3. When done, press "Cancel" button and release the pressure naturally.
4. Open the pot and serve warm.
5. Enjoy!

301. Curried Carrot Kale Soup

Preparation Time: 40 Minutes
Servings: 2
Ingredients:

- 2 cups kale, finely chopped (frozen or fresh
- 8 carrots, chopped
- 5 potatoes, chopped
- ½ yellow onion, chopped
- 3 garlic cloves, minced
- ¼ cup peanut butter, powdered
- 1 tsp cayenne pepper
- 1 tbsp curry powder
- 4 cups water
- 2 tsp of vegetable base (or use 2 cups water with 2 cups veggie broth

Directions:

1. Add garlic and onion to Instant Pot along with ¼ cup water and Switch on

'Sautée' button. Sauté garlic and onions for 5 minutes.

2. Add peanut butter, cayenne and curry powder and stir. Add bit water if needed. Sauté this for 2 more minutes.

3. Except for the kale, add remaining ingredients, cover with lid and switch on manual button for 8 minutes on high pressure.

4. When timer beeps, allow natural pressure release for 10-15 minutes. Set steam release handle to 'venting'. Open the lid.

5. Using an immersion blender, blend the soup until desired consistency.

6. Add chopped kale and stir again.

302. Italian Plum Tomato Soup

Preparation Time: 10 Minutes
Servings: 6
Ingredients:
- 1 (28-ouncecan Italian plum tomatoes
- ½ cup nondairy milk
- 1 large yellow onion, chopped
- 1 teaspoon dried marjoram
- 1 (14-ouncecan crushed tomatoes
- 1 cup vegetable broth
- 2 tablespoons tomato paste
- 1 teaspoon dried basil
- 1 teaspoon brown sugar
- ¼ cup oil-packed sun-dried tomatoes, chopped
- 2 garlic cloves, minced
- Salt and freshly ground black pepper

Directions:
1. In an instant pot add the oil with garlic, onion and tomato paste.

2. Cooking Time: for 1 minute and add the marjoram, basil, brown sugar and Cooking Time: for another minute.

3. Add the rest of the ingredients and

mix well.

4. Add the lid and Cooking Time: for about 5 minutes.

5. Transfer the mix to a blender.

6. Blend until smooth and serve warm.

303. Balsamic Hatchet Soup

Preparation Time: 20 Minutes
Servings: 4
A hatchet soup is one where you combine any number of different ingredients, and is great for using up a medley of vegetables.
Ingredients:
- 3 shallots, halved
- 3 garlic cloves, minced
- 6 ounces green beans, trimmed and halved
- 1 red or yellow bell pepper, seeded and cut into ¼-inch strips
- 8 ounces mushrooms, halved, quartered, or sliced
- 3 small zucchini, halved lengthwise and cut into ¼-inch slices
- 2 small yellow summer squash, halved lengthwise and cut into ¼-inch slices
- 1½ cups cherry tomatoes, halved
- ½ cup balsamic reduction
- 3 tablespoons chopped fresh basil
- 2 tablespoons chopped fresh flat-leaf parsley
- 2 teaspoons olive oil
- Salt and freshly ground black pepper

Directions:
1. Put the oil in your instant pot and warm.

2. Add the shallots and soften for 3 minutes.

3. Add the garlic and Cooking Time: another minute.

4. Add the green beans, bell pepper, mushrooms, zucchini, and yellow

squash.

5. Seal and Cooking Time: on Stew for 10 minutes.
6. Depressurize quickly, add the tomato, basil, and parsley.
7. Reseal and Cooking Time: on Stew 2 minutes.
8. Depressurize naturally and serve drizzled with balsamic reduction.

304. Pearl Barley Tomato Mushroom Soup

Preparation Time: 6 Minutes
Servings: 6
Ingredients:

- 1(14-ouncecan crushed tomatoes
- ½cup pearl barley
- ½ounce dried porcini mushrooms, rinsed
- 1ounces cremini mushrooms, sliced
- 2teaspoons olive oil (optional
- 1large carrot, chopped
- 5cups vegetable broth
- 1large yellow onion, chopped
- Salt and freshly ground black pepper
- 1teaspoon dried thyme
- 4ounces shiitake mushrooms, stemmed and sliced
- 2tablespoons soy sauce

Directions:

1. Add the oil in your instant pot.
2. Toss the onion and make it caramelized.
3. Add the remaining ingredients.
4. Mix well and Cooking Time: for 5 minutes with the lid on.
5. Serve warm.

305. Sweet Potato Soup

Preparation Time: 20 Minutes
Servings: 2
Ingredients:

- 2 large sweet potatoes, peeled and chopped
- 1 medium carrot, sliced
- 1 medium onion, finely chopped
- 2 cups vegetable broth
- 2 garlic cloves, finely chopped
- 1 tsp salt
- ½ tsp black pepper, freshly ground
- 1 tbsp olive oil

Directions:

1. Plug in your instant pot and press "Sautee" button. Grease the stainless steel insert and add potatoes, onions, and garlic. Stir-fry for 3-4 minutes, or until onions translucent.
2. Now, add the remaining ingredients and stir well until combined. Close the lid and adjust the steam release handle. Press "Manual" button and set the timer for 7 minutes. Cooking Time: on high pressure.
3. When done, press "Cancel" button and perform a quick release. Let it stand for 10 minutes before opening.
4. Enjoy!

306. Corn Chowder

Preparation Time: 5 Minutes
Servings: 4
Ingredients:

- 4cups fresh corn kernels
- 1onion, chopped
- 2chipotle chilies in adobo, minced
- Salt and black pepper
- 1celery rib, chopped
- 4cups vegetable broth

- 1Potato, peeled and diced

Directions:

1. Add the corn kernels, onion, chiles in adobo, seasoning, celery rib, and potato in your instant pot.
2. Pour in the broth and mix well.
3. Cooking Time: for 10 minutes.
4. Use a hand blender to blend the mixture.
5. Serve warm.

307. Onion Soup

Preparation Time: 5 Minutes
Servings: 6
Ingredients:

- 4slices French or Italian bread, cubed
- 1teaspoon vegan Worcestershire sauce
- 2tablespoons olive oil
- ½teaspoon dried thyme
- 5cups vegetable broth
- 5onions, sliced
- Salt and black pepper

Directions:

1. Add the oil in your instant pot.
2. Add the onion and toss for 30 seconds.
3. Add the rest of the ingredients.
4. Cover and Cooking Time: for about 3 minutes.
5. Serve hot.

308. Baby Spinach Coconut Soup

Preparation Time: 5 Minutes
Servings: 4
Ingredients:

- 2jalapeños, seeded and minced
- 8ounces baby spinach
- 1onion, chopped
- ½teaspoon fresh thyme
- 3garlic cloves, chopped

- 1red bell pepper, seeded and chopped
- 4cups vegetable broth
- ¼teaspoon ground allspice
- Salt and black pepper
- 1(14.5-ouncecan diced tomatoes, drained
- 1(13.5-ouncecan coconut milk
- 1½cups cooked dark red kidney beans
- 2potatoes, peeled and diced

Directions:

1. Toss the garlic and onion in an instant pot for 30 seconds.
2. Add the vegetables, kidney beans, coconut milk, broth, spices, and herbs.
3. Mix well and Cooking Time: for 4 minutes with the lid on.
4. Serve hot.

309. Cabbage Carrot Beet Soup

Preparation Time: 10 Minutes
Servings: 6
Ingredients:

- 1carrot, shredded
- 5cups vegetable broth
- 2tablespoons fresh lemon juice
- ¼cup minced fresh dill
- 1teaspoon light brown sugar
- ½teaspoon caraway seeds
- 1onion, minced
- 1Potato, peeled and minced
- Salt and black pepper
- 3cups shredded cabbage
- 4beets, peeled and minced
- 1teaspoon dried thyme

Directions:

1. Add the cabbage, carrot, potato, beets in your instant pot.
2. Add the sugar, dill, and the rest of the ingredients.
3. Cooking Time: for 6 minutes with the

lid on.

4. Serve hot.

310. Tomato Tortilla Soup

Preparation Time: 5 Minutes
Servings: 4
Ingredients:

- 1jalapeño chile, seeded and minced
- 1onion, minced
- ½cup chopped fresh cilantro leaves
- 2tablespoons tomato paste
- 3cups lightly crushed tortilla chips
- 3garlic cloves, minced
- 1(14-ouncecan diced tomatoes
- 1teaspoon ground cumin
- 5cups vegetable broth
- Salt and black pepper
- 3teaspoons chipotle chiles in adobo, minced

Directions:

1. Add all the ingredients in an instant pot except the chips.
2. Cover and Cooking Time: for 3 minutes.
3. Add the chips and Cooking Time: for another 2 minutes.
4. Serve hot.

311. Basil Marjoram Tomato Soup

Preparation Time: 10 Minutes
Servings: 6
Ingredients:

- ¼cup oil-packed sun-dried tomatoes, chopped
- 1(28-ouncecan tomatoes
- 1teaspoon dried marjoram
- 2teaspoons olive oil (optional
- 2tablespoons tomato paste
- 2garlic cloves, minced

- 1teaspoon dried basil
- 1 cup vegetable broth
- 1(14-ouncecan crushed tomatoes
- 1onion, chopped
- 1teaspoon brown sugar
- Salt and black pepper

Directions:

1. In your instant pot add all the ingredients one by one.
2. Mix well using a wooden spoon.
3. Cooking Time: for 10 Minutes with the lid on.
4. Add the mixture to a blender and blend until smooth.
5. Serve hot.

312. Porcini Mushroom And Barley Soup

Preparation Time: 10 Minutes
Servings: 6
Ingredients:

- 4ounces shiitake mushrooms, stemmed and sliced
- ½cup pearl barley
- ½ounce dried porcini mushrooms, rinsed
- 1onion, chopped
- 1(14-ouncecan crushed tomatoes
- 1large carrot, chopped
- 1teaspoon dried thyme
- 5cups vegetable broth
- 8ounces mushrooms, sliced
- 2tablespoons soy sauce
- 2teaspoons olive oil (optional
- Salt and black pepper

Directions:

1. In your instant pot add the mushroom, broth, seasoning, herbs, spices, and vegetables.
2. Add the pearl barley and mix well.

150

3. Cover with lid and Cooking Time: for about 8 minutes.
4. Serve hot.

313. Tofu Mushroom Kombu Soup

Preparation Time: 10 Minutes
Servings: 4
Ingredients:

- 1pound cabbage, thinly sliced
- 8ounces extra-firm tofu, cut into ½-inch dice
- 4cups water
- 4ounces shiitake mushrooms, sliced
- 1(1-inchpiece peeled fresh ginger
- ½cup soy sauce
- 1ounce enoki mushrooms, trimmed
- 1(3-inchpiece kombu sea vegetable
- 1bunch scallions, sliced
- 2ounces cellophane noodles
- ½cup mirin
- 1carrot, sliced
- Salt
- 8ounces seitan, sliced

Directions:

1. In your instant pot add ginger, water, soy sauce, kombu, and mirin.
2. Mix well and Cooking Time: for 2 minutes.
3. Discard the ginger and kombu and add the rest of the ingredients.
4. Mix well and cover with lid.
5. Cooking Time: for 5 minutes with the lid on.
6. Use a hand blender to blend well.
7. Serve hot.

314. Basmati Rice Coconut Milk Soup

Preparation Time: 10 Minutes
Servings: 6
Ingredients:

- 3cups cooked brown basmati rice
- 1sweet potato, peeled and diced
- 1(13-ouncecan coconut milk
- 1red bell pepper, seeded and chopped
- 1onion, chopped
- 4cups vegetable broth
- 1tablespoon curry powder
- ½teaspoon cayenne pepper, or to taste
- 3garlic cloves, minced
- 1½cups cooked chickpeas
- 2teaspoons grated fresh ginger
- 1teaspoon ground coriander
- 1Apple, peeled, cored, and chopped
- 2tablespoons fresh lemon juice
- Salt and black pepper
- 1green bell pepper, seeded and chopped

Directions:

1. In your instant pot add the ginger, garlic and onion and toss for a minute.
2. Add the spices, and vegetables. Add the rest of the ingredients and stir well.
3. Cover and Cooking Time: for about 5 minutes.
4. Transfer the mixture to a blender and blend until smooth.
5. Serve hot.

315. Rice Noodle Soup

Preparation Time: 10 Minutes
Servings: 4
Ingredients:

- 8ounces dried rice noodles
- 6cups vegetable broth
- 1½tablespoons fresh lime juice
- 3whole cloves
- 2tablespoons barley miso paste
- 3whole star anise
- 1fresh ginger, minced
- 1small yellow onion, minced
- 3garlic cloves, minced
- 6ounces seitan, sliced
- 3tablespoons hoisin sauce
- 3tablespoons soy sauce

Directions:

1. In a cloth add the ginger, cloves, star anise and tie it tightly.
2. Add all the ingredients in your instant pot.
3. Add the ginger cloth to the pot.
4. Cover with lid and Cooking Time: for 7 minutes.
5. Discard the ginger cloth and serve hot.

316. Indian Red Split Lentil Soup

Preparation Time: 5 Minutes
Cooking Time: 50 Minutes
Servings: 4

Ingredients

- 1 cup red split lentils
- 2 cups water
- 1 teaspoon curry powder plus 1 tablespoon, divided, or 5 coriander seeds (optional
- 1 teaspoon coconut oil, or 1 tablespoon water or vegetable broth
- 1 red onion, diced
- 1 tablespoon minced fresh ginger
- 2 cups peeled and cubed sweet potato
- 1 cup sliced zucchini
- Freshly ground black pepper
- Sea salt
- 3 to 4 cups vegetable stock, or water
- 1 to 2 teaspoons toasted sesame oil
- 1 bunch spinach, chopped
- Toasted sesame seeds

Directions

1. Preparing the Ingredients.
2. Put the lentils in a large pot with 2 cups water, and 1 teaspoon of the curry powder. Bring the lentils to a boil, then reduce the heat and simmer, covered, for about 10 minutes, until the lentils are soft.
3. Meanwhile, heat a large pot over medium heat. Add the coconut oil and sauté the onion and ginger until soft, about 5 minutes. Add the sweet potato and leave it on the heat about 10 minutes to soften slightly, then add the zucchini and Cooking Time: until it starts to look shiny, about 5 minutes. Add the remaining 1 tablespoon curry powder, pepper, and salt, and stir the vegetables to coat.
4. Add the vegetable stock, bring to a boil, then turn down to simmer and cover. Let the vegetables slowly Cooking Time: for 20 to 30 minutes, or until the sweet potato is tender.
5. Add the fully cooked lentils to the soup. Add another pinch salt, the toasted sesame oil, and the spinach. Stir, allowing the spinach to wilt before removing the pot from the heat.
6. Serve garnished with toasted sesame seeds.

Nutrition: Calories: 319; Protein: 16g; Total fat: 8g; Carbohydrates: 50g; Fiber: 10g

317. Light Vegetable Broth

Preparation Time: 10 Minutes
Cooking Time: Time:1 Hour 30 Minutes
Servings: About 6 Cups

Ingredients

- 1 tablespoon olive oil
- 2 medium onions, quartered
- 2 medium carrots, chopped
- 1 celery rib, chopped
- 2 garlic cloves, unpeeled and crushed
- 8 cups water
- 2 teaspoons soy sauce
- 1/3 cup coarsely chopped fresh parsley
- 1 bay leaf
- 1 teaspoon salt
- 1/2 teaspoon black peppercorns

Directions

1. In a large stockpot, heat the oil over medium heat. Add the onions, carrots, celery, and garlic. Cover and Cooking Time: until softened, about 10 minutes. Stir in the water, soy sauce, parsley, bay leaf, salt, and peppercorns. Bring to a boil and then reduce heat to low and simmer, uncovered, for 11/2 hours.
2. Set aside to cool, then strain through a fine-mesh sieve into a large bowl or pot, pressing against the solids with the back of a spoon to release all the liquid. Discard solids. Cool broth completely, then portion into tightly covered containers and refrigerate for up to 4 days or freeze for up to 3 months.

318. Roasted Vegetable Broth

Preparation Time: 5 Minutes
Cooking Time: 1hour 30 Minutes •
Servings: About 6 Cups

Ingredients

- 1 large onion, thickly sliced
- 2 large carrots, chopped
- 1 celery rib, chopped
- 1 large potato, unpeeled and chopped
- 3 garlic cloves, unpeeled and crushed
- 2 tablespoons olive oil
- Salt and freshly ground black pepper
- 8 cups water
- 1/2 cup coarsely chopped fresh parsley
- 2 bay leaves
- 1/2 teaspoon black peppercorns
- 1 tablespoon soy sauce

Directions

1. Preheat the oven to 425°F. In a lightly oiled 9 x 13-inch baking pan, place the onion, carrots, celery, potato, and garlic. Drizzle with the oil and sprinkle with salt and pepper to taste. Roast the vegetables until they are slightly browned, turning once, about 30 minutes total. Set aside for 10 minutes to cool slightly.
2. Place the roasted vegetables in a large stockpot. Add the water, parsley, bay leaves, peppercorns, soy sauce, and salt to taste. Bring to a boil and then reduce heat to low and simmer, uncovered, until the broth has reduced slightly and is a deep golden color, about 1 hour.
3. Set aside to cool, then strain through a fine-mesh sieve into a large bowl or pot, pressing against the solids with the back of a spoon to release all the liquid. Discard solids. Cool broth completely, then portion into tightly

covered containers and refrigerate for up to 4 days or freeze for up to 3 months.

319. Root Vegetable Broth

Preparation Time: 5 Minutes • Cooking Time: Time:1 Hour 38 Minutes •
Servings: About 6 Cups

Ingredients

- 1 tablespoon olive oil
- 1 large onion, coarsely chopped
- 2 medium carrots, coarsely chopped
- 2 medium parsnips, coarsely chopped
- 1 medium turnip, coarsely chopped
- 8 cups water
- 1 medium white potato, unpeeled and quartered
- 3 garlic cloves, unpeeled and crushed
- ¾ cup coarsely chopped fresh parsley
- 2 bay leaves
- 1/2 teaspoon black peppercorns
- 1 teaspoon salt

Directions

1. In a large stockpot, heat the oil over medium heat. Add the onion, carrots, parsnips, and turnip. Cover and Cooking Time: until softened, about 8 minutes. Stir in the water. Add the potato, garlic, parsley, bay leaves, peppercorns, and salt. Bring to a boil and then reduce heat to low and simmer, uncovered, for 11/2 hours.
2. Set aside to cool, then strain through a fine-mesh sieve into a large bowl or pot, pressing against the solids with the back of a spoon to release all the liquid. Discard solids. Cool broth completely, then portion into tightly covered containers and refrigerate for up to 4 days or freeze for up to 3 months.

320. Mushroom Vegetable Broth

Preparation Time: 5 Minutes • Cooking Time: Time:1 Hour 37 Minutes •
Servings: About 6 Cups

Ingredients

- 1 tablespoon olive oil
- 1 medium onion, unpeeled and quartered
- 1 medium carrot, coarsely chopped
- 1 celery rib with leaves, coarsely chopped
- 8 ounces white mushrooms, lightly rinsed, patted dry, and coarsely chopped
- 5 dried shiitake or porcini mushrooms, soaked in 2 cups hot water, drained, soaking liquid strained and reserved
- 3 garlic cloves, unpeeled and crushed
- 1/2 cup coarsely chopped fresh parsley
- 2 bay leaves
- 1/2 teaspoon black peppercorns
- 1 teaspoon salt
- 5 cups water

Directions

1. In a large stockpot, heat the oil over medium heat. Add the onion, carrot, celery, and white mushrooms. Cover and Cooking Time: until softened, about 7 minutes. Stir in the softened dried mushrooms and the reserved soaking liquid, along with the garlic, parsley, bay leaves, peppercorns, salt, and water. Bring to a boil and then reduce heat to low and simmer, uncovered, for 11/2 hours.
2. Set aside to cool, then strain through a fine-mesh sieve into a large bowl or pot, pressing against the solids with the back of a spoon to release all the

liquid. Discard solids. Cool broth completely, then portion into tightly covered containers and refrigerate for up to 4 days or freeze for up to 3 months.

321. Jamaican Red Bean Stew

Preparation Time: 10 Minutes
Cooking Time: 40 Minutes
Servings: 4

Ingredients

- 1 tablespoon olive oil
- 1 medium yellow onion, chopped
- 2 large carrots, cut into 1/4-inch slices
- 2 garlic cloves, minced
- 1 large sweet potato, peeled and cut into 1/4-inch dice
- 1/4 teaspoon crushed red pepper
- 3 cups cooked or 2 (15.5-ouncecans dark red kidney beans, drained and rinsed
- 1 (14.5-ouncecan diced tomatoes, drained
- 1 teaspoon hot or mild curry powder
- 1 teaspoon dried thyme
- 1/4 teaspoon ground allspice
- 1/2 teaspoon salt
- 1/4 teaspoon freshly ground black pepper
- 1/2 cup water
- 1 (13.5-ouncecan unsweetened coconut milk

Directions

1. In a large saucepan, heat the oil over medium heat. Add the onion and carrots, cover, and Cooking Time: until softened, 5 minutes.
2. Add the garlic, sweet potato, and crushed red pepper. Stir in the kidney beans, tomatoes, curry powder, thyme, allspice, salt, and black pepper.

3. Stir in the water, cover, and simmer until the vegetables are tender, about 30 minutes. Stir in the coconut milk and simmer, uncovered, for 10 minutes to blend flavors and thicken the sauce. If a thicker sauce is desired, puree some of the vegetables with an immersion blender. Serve immediately.

322. Greens And Beans Soup

Preparation Time: 15 Minutes
Cooking Time: 0 Minutes
Servings: 4

Ingredients

- 1 tablespoon olive oil
- 1 medium onion, chopped
- 3 large garlic cloves, minced
- 11/2 cups cooked or 1 (15.5-ouncecan cannellini beans, drained and rinsed
- 11/2 cups cooked or 1 (15.5-ouncecan dark red kidney beans, drained and rinsed
- 5 cups vegetable broth, homemade (see Light Vegetable Brothor store-bought, or water
- 1/4 teaspoon crushed red pepper
- Salt and freshly ground black pepper
- 3 cups coarsely chopped stemmed Swiss chard
- 3 cups coarsely chopped stemmed kale

Directions

1. In a large soup pot, heat the oil over medium heat. Add the onion, cover, and Cooking Time: until softened, about 5 minutes. Add the garlic and cook, uncovered, 1 minute.
2. Stir in the beans, broth, crushed red pepper, and salt and black pepper to taste and bring to a boil. Reduce heat to a simmer, uncovered, and stir in the

greens. Continue to Cooking Time: until the greens are tender, 15 to 20 minutes. Serve hot.

323. Hearty Chili

Preparation Time: 10 Minutes
Cooking Time: 15 Minutes
Servings: 4

Ingredients

- 1 onion, diced
- 2 to 3 garlic cloves, minced
- 1 teaspoon olive oil, or 1 to 2 tablespoons water, vegetable broth, or red wine
- 1 (28-ouncecan tomatoes
- ¼ cup tomato paste, or crushed tomatoes
- 1 (14-ouncecan kidney beans, rinsed and drained, or 1½ cups cooked
- 2 to 3 teaspoons chili powder
- ¼ teaspoon sea salt
- ¼ cup fresh cilantro, or parsley leaves

Directions

1. Preparing the Ingredients.
2. In a large pot, sauté the onion and garlic in the oil, about 5 minutes. Once they're soft, add the tomatoes, tomato paste, beans, and chili powder. Season with the salt.
3. Let simmer for at least 10 minutes, or as long as you like. The flavors will get better the longer it simmers, and it's even better as leftovers.
4. Garnish with cilantro and serve.

Nutrition: Calories: 160; Protein: 8g; Total fat: 3g; Saturated fat: 11g; Carbohydrates: 29g; Fiber: 7g

324. Golden Beet Soup With A Twist

Preparation Time: 5 Minutes
Cooking Time: 50 Minutes
Servings: 6

Ingredients

- 2 tablespoons olive oil
- 1 medium yellow onion, finely chopped
- 1 medium carrot, finely chopped
- 4 medium golden beets, peeled and diced
- 1 small yellow bell pepper, chopped
- 1 medium Yukon Gold potato, diced
- 5 cups vegetable broth, homemade (see Light Vegetable Brothor store-bought, or water
- 1 teaspoon dried thyme
- Salt and freshly ground black pepper
- 1 tablespoon fresh lemon juice
- 2 tablespoons minced fresh dillweed or 11/2 teaspoons dried, for garnish

Directions

1. In a large soup pot, heat the oil over medium heat. Add the onion and carrot. Cover and Cooking Time: until softened, 5 minutes. Add the beets, bell pepper, and potato and cook, uncovered, stirring, for 1 minute. Stir in the broth, sugar, and thyme and season with salt and black pepper to taste. Cooking Time: until the vegetables are tender, about 45 minutes.
2. Serve hot or, alternately, set aside to cool, then refrigerate until chilled. Just before serving, stir in the lemon juice and garnish with the dill.

325. Asian-Inspired Chili

Preparation Time: 15 Minutes
Cooking Time: 20 Minutes
Servings: 4

Ingredients

- 1 teaspoon sesame oil or 2 teaspoons vegetable broth or water
- 1 cup diced onion
- 3 teaspoons minced garlic (about 3 cloves
- 1 cup chopped carrots
- 2 cups shredded green or napa cabbage
- 1 (14.5-ouncecan small red beans or adzuki beans, drained and rinsed
- 1 (14.5-ouncefire-roasted diced tomatoes
- 2 cups vegetable broth
- 2 tablespoons red miso paste or tomato paste
- 2 tablespoons hot water
- 1 tablespoon hot sauce
- 2 teaspoons to 1 tablespoon tamari or soy sauce (optional

Directions

1. Preparing the Ingredients.
2. In a large pot, over medium-high heat, heat the sesame oil. Add the onion, garlic, and carrot. Sauté for 5 minutes, until the onions are translucent. Add the cabbage, beans, tomatoes, and broth, and stir well. Bring to a boil.
3. Cover, reduce the heat to low, and simmer for 15 minutes.
4. In a measuring cup, whisk the miso paste and hot water. Set aside.
5. After 15 minutes, remove the chili from the stove, add the miso mixture and hot sauce, and stir well. Taste before determining how much tamari to add (if using).
6. Divide the chili evenly among 4 single-serving containers or large glass jars. Let cool before sealing the lids.
7. Place the containers in the refrigerator for up to 5 days or freeze for up to 3 months. To thaw, refrigerate overnight. Reheat in the microwave for 2 to 3 minutes.

Nutrition: Calories: 177; Protein: 9g; Total fat: 2g; Carbohydrates: 33g; Fiber: 191g

PASTA

326. 5-Ingredients Pasta

Preparation Time: 25 minutes
Servings: 6

Ingredients

- Dry pasta: 1 pound
- Different vegetables: 1 pound (tomatoes, zucchini, and red onion
- Vegan marinara sauce: 125 oz. jar
- Hummus: ¼ cup
- Olive oil
- Salt: as per your need

Directions:

1. Preheat the oven to 400F
2. Add water and salt to the pot and boil and Cooking Time: pasta as per packet instruction
3. Chop all the vegetables and spread on the baking sheet and brush with olive oil and salt
4. Roast the vegetables for 15 minutes
5. Prepare the sauce by combining hummus and marinara sauce together in a pan and put on medium heat
6. Add vegetables and pasta to the sauce and combine well
7. Serve warm

Nutrition:
Carbs: 65 g
Protein: 14 g
Fats: 2 g
Calories: 329 Kcal

327. Brussels Sprout Penne

Preparation Time: 20 minutes
Servings: 2

Ingredients

- Penne: 1 cup
- Brussels Sprout: 320g roasted halved
- Garlic: 2 cloves thinly sliced
- Olive oil: 2 tbsp
- Chili flakes: 1 tsp
- Salt: as per your taste
- Pepper: as per your taste
- Lemon: 1 juice and zest

Directions:

1. Cooking Time: the pasta as per the packet instruction
2. Take a large pan and heat oil
3. Add in garlic and Cooking Time: for two minutes
4. Add in chili flakes and Cooking Time: for a minutes
5. Add pasta, lemon juice and zest, salt, pepper, and roasted Brussels sprouts
6. Mix everything well and serve

Nutrition:
Carbs:24.7 g
Protein:5.75 g
Fats:14.9 g
Calories: 245Kcal

328. Bang Bang Sauce With Pasta

Preparation Time: 40 minutes
Servings: 4

Ingredients

- Pasta: 4 cups cooked

For the cauliflower:

- Cauliflower:1 head diced
- Rice crisp cereal:3 cups
- Rice flour:1/4 cup
- Garlic powder:1/4 tsp
- Ground black pepper:1/4 tsp
- Salt:1/4 tsp
- Neutral oil:1 tbsp
- Water:6 tbsp

For the bang bang sauce:

- Vegan mayonnaise:1/4 cup
- Rice vinegar:1 tsp
- Sweet chili sauce:3 tbsp
- Hot sauce:1 tbsp

Directions:

1. Cooking Time: pasta as per packet instruction
2. Preheat the oven to 400F
3. Line parchment paper on the baking sheet and spray with oil
4. Make crumbs of the rice crisp cereal by pulsing in the food processor
5. Mix the crumbs with black pepper, garlic powder, and salt
6. Make a thin batter of the rice flour using water
7. Now take a single cauliflower floret and dip in the rice flour mixture
8. Then add it to the cereal crumbs to coat it
9. Place them to the baking sheet one by one
10. Oil spray from the top and bake for 25 minutes
11. Add all the sauce ingredients and mix well
12. Serve the sauce and cauliflower together with pasta

Nutrition:

Carbs: 97 g

Protein: 13.5g

Fats: 5.6 g

Calories: 497 Kcal

329. Beans And Pasta

Preparation Time: 30 minutes

Servings: 2

Ingredients

- Pasta: 1 cup cooked
- Beans: 1 cup rinsed and drained well
- Onion: 1 cup finely diced

- Tomato: 2 cups diced
- Lemon juice: 2 tbsp
- Harissa 2 tsp
- Olive oil: 2 tbsp
- Fresh coriander: 2 tbsp chopped
- Garlic: 1 clove crushed

Directions:

1. Cooking Time: pasta as per packet instructions
2. Add garlic, lemon juice, harissa, and olive oil in a bowl and whisk
3. Take a serving bowl and combine pasta, beans, onion, tomatoes, and the sauce you made
4. Add fresh coriander from the top and serve

Nutrition:

Carbs: 64.3g

Protein: 16.5

Fats: 20.6

Calories: 459Kcal

330. Broccoli Elbow Macaroni

Preparation Time: 40 minutes

Servings: 2

Ingredients

- Elbow macaroni: 1 cup (after cooked
- Broccoli florets: 1 cup
- Spinach: 1 cup chopped
- Onion: 1 chopped
- Garlic: 2 tsp paste
- Ginger: 2 tsp paste
- Cumin: 1 tsp
- Cayenne pepper: ¼ tsp
- Cooking oil: 2 tbsp
- Dried oregano: ½ tsp
- Salt and pepper: as per your taste
- Cilantro: 2 tbsp
- Almond milk: ¼ cup

- Water: as per your need

Directions:

1. Take a saucepan and heat oil in it
2. Add garlic, ginger, and onion to it and make them tender
3. Add salt, cayenne pepper, cumin, and pepper and bring to boil
4. Now add broccoli florets and spinach and mix for a minute
5. Lower the heat to medium and Cooking Time: for 10 minutes
6. In the meanwhile, Cooking Time: elbow macaroni as per packet instructions
7. Add macaroni to the broccoli pan and mix well
8. Add almond milk from the top and mix well
9. Remove from heat and add to the serving bowl
10. Garnish with cilantro and sprinkle oregano from the top and serve

Nutrition:
Carbs: 34.15g
Protein: 8.8g
Fats: 11.3g
Calories: 232Kcal

331. Broccoli Pasta

Preparation Time: 45 minutes
Servings: 2

Ingredients

- Pasta: 1 cup cooked
- Broccoli: 2 cups cut in big florets
- Hot sauce: 2 tbsp
- Rice vinegar: 1 tbsp
- Salt: as per your taste
- Pepper: as per your taste
- Sliced red pepper: 1 cup sliced
- Olive oil: 1 tbsp

Directions:

1. Cooking Time: pasta as per packet instruction
2. Preheat the oven 200C
3. Add broccoli to the baking sheet and sprinkle seasoning and brush with olive oil
4. Roast for 25 minutes till it turns golden and soft
5. Take a small bowl and combine hot sauce, vinegar, salt, and pepper
6. Remove broccoli from oven and brush with this dressing and Cooking Time: in the oven again for 10 minutes
7. Add to the serving bowl and serve with red pepper
8. Serve at the top of pasta

Nutrition:
Carbs: 28.5 g
Protein: 6.6g
Fats: 8.5g
Calories: 223Kcal

332. Caponata Pasta

Preparation Time: 55 minutes
Servings: 4

Ingredients

- Wholewheat spaghetti: 300g
- Aubergines: 2 cut into 3cm cubes
- Red onion: ½ sliced
- Vegetable oi:l 4 tsp
- Raisins: 2 tbsp heaped
- Celery: 2 sticks sliced
- Garlic: 2 cloves sliced
- Dried oregano:1 tsp
- Chopped tomatoes:400g tin
- Capers: 1 tsp
- Vinegar: 2 tbsp
- Kalamata olives: a handful chopped
- Flat-leaf parsley a small bunch,

chopped

Directions:

1. Preheat the oven to 200C
2. Take a bowl and add 2 tablespoons oil and seasoning and add the aubergine
3. Place them to the baking sheet and Cooking Time: for 20 minutes
4. Take a large pan and heat the remaining oil
5. Add in celery, red onion, and salt and Cooking Time: for 10 minutes
6. Add oregano and garlic and stir and then add tomatoes and 100ml water
7. Add in aubergine and Cooking Time: for 15 minutes and allow the sauce to thicken
8. Add vinegar, capers, and raisins and lower the heat
9. Cooking Time: the pasta as per packet instruction and drain
10. Add pasta to the caponata and top with parsley
11. Mix well and serve

Nutrition:

Carbs: 61g

Protein: 13.8g

Fats: 6.7g

Calories: 387Kcal

333. Carbonara With Pine Nuts

Preparation Time: 45 minutes

Servings: 6

Ingredients

- Spaghetti: 450g
- Cauliflower: 1 small with leaves separated and reserved
- Salt: as per your taste
- Garlic 2 cloves, peeled
- White pepper
- Olive oil: 3 tbsp
- Vegetable stock: 750ml

- Pine nuts: 4 tbsp toasted

Directions:

1. Preheat the oven to 200C
2. Take a bowl and add 1 tablespoon oil and seasoning and add cauliflower leaves
3. Place them to the baking sheet and Cooking Time: for 12 minutes
4. Break the cauliflower and separate florets and stalk
5. Take a pan and add the stock, garlic, and 2 tablespoons oil and add the cauliflower
6. Cover and Cooking Time: for 20 minutes
7. Remove cauliflower and garlic from the pan and blend together
8. Make the sauce by adding a small amount of water
9. Add back to the pan and mix in salt and pepper
10. Cooking Time: pasta and add to the sauce
11. Serve with pine nuts and cauliflower leaves on the top

Nutrition:

Carbs: 61.4g

Protein: 13.7g

Fats: 14.4g

Calories: 441Kcal

334. Casarecce With Raw Tomato Sauce

Preparation Time: 15 minutes

Servings: 2

Ingredients

- Casarecce: 200g
- Cherry tomatoes: 250g, halved
- Spring onions: 3 chopped
- Vinegar: 3 tbsp
- Olive oil: 4 tbsp

- Tabasco: 4-5 dashes
- Salt: as per your taste
- Pepper: as per your taste
- Basil: 2 tbsp torn

Directions:
1. Take a bowl and add in cherry tomatoes, olive oil, vinegar, Tabasco, spring onion, and a lot of salt and pepper
2. Cooking Time: casarecce as per packet instructions
3. Drain the pasta but keep 2 tablespoons of water and add to the sauce
4. Add pasta to the sauce
5. Top with torn basil and serve

Nutrition:
Carbs: 74.8g
Protein: 14.5g
Fats: 24.3g
Calories: 595Kcal

335. Cauli Cabbage Pasta

Preparation Time: 30 minutes
Servings: 4

Ingredients
- Pasta: 2 cups (after cooked
- Olive oil: 1 tbsp
- Cauliflower: 2 cups diced
- Garlic: 3 cloves minced
- Red onion: 1 small diced
- Cabbage: 1 cup diced
- Soy sauce: 1 tbsp
- Salt: 1 tsp
- Black pepper: ½ tsp
- Green onions: 2 tbsp

Directions:
1. Cooking Time: pasta as per packet instructions
2. Take a large saucepan and add olive

oil and heat on medium flame
3. Include onion and garlic to the pan and Cooking Time: for a minute
4. Now add cabbage, cabbage, salt, pepper, and soy sauce and stir for 5 minutes
5. Then add cooked pasta and mix well
6. Then cover and Cooking Time: for 2 minutes on low flame and remove from heat
7. Sprinkle green onion on top and serve

Nutrition:
Carbs: 22.6g
Protein: 5.2g
Fats: 4.4g
Calories: 148Kcal

336. Chickpeas Pasta

Preparation Time: 30 minutes
Servings: 4

Ingredients
- Pasta: 1 ½ cup (after cooking
- Olive oil: 2 tbsp
- Garlic: 2 cloves minced
- Chickpeas: 1 cup can
- Red onion: 1 small diced
- Bell pepper: 1 cup diced
- Zucchini: 1 cup diced
- Tomatoes: 1 cup diced
- Chili powder: 1 tsp
- Cumin: 1 tsp
- Salt: 1 tsp
- Black pepper: ½ tsp
- Green onions: 2 tbsp chopped

Directions:
1. Cooking Time: pasta as per packet instructions
2. Take a large saucepan and add olive oil and heat on medium flame
3. Include onion and garlic to the pan

and Cooking Time: for a minute

4. Now add bell pepper, zucchini, tomatoes, chickpeas, cumin, salt, pepper, and chili powder and stir
5. Cooking Time: for 10 minutes
6. Stir the spoon and add cooked pasta
7. Then cover and Cooking Time: for 5 minutes on low flame and remove from heat
8. Sprinkle green onion on top and serve

Nutrition:
Carbs: 36g
Protein: 9.8g
Fats: 5.9g
Calories: 234Kcal

337. Chili Pasta With Chickpeas Gravy

Preparation Time: 30 minutes
Servings: 4

Ingredients

- Pasta: 2 cups (after cooking
- Olive oil: 2 tbsp
- Jalapeño: 1 diced
- Green chili: 2 finely diced
- Salt: as per your need
- Garlic: 2 cloves minced
- Red onion: 1 small diced
- Dried oregano: 2 tbsp
- For the gravy:
- Vegetable oil 2 tsp
- Chickpeas: 1 cup rinsed and drained
- Onions: 2 thinly sliced
- Plain flour 1 tbsp
- Water: 250 ml
- Boiled water: 600 ml
- Vegan gravy granules: 2 tbsp

Directions:
1. Cooking Time: pasta as per packet instructions
2. Take a large saucepan and add olive oil and heat on medium flame
3. Include onion and garlic to the pan and Cooking Time: for a minute
4. Add pasta, chili, and jalapeño and sprinkle salt and mix well
5. For the gravy, take a pan and heat oil
6. Add in onions and stir then add salt and water
7. Allow the water to evaporate so that onion caramelized
8. Add in flour and Cooking Time: for a minute and then add gravy granules and boiled water
9. Cooking Time: till the gravy becomes thick and then add chickpeas and simmer for 5 minutes
10. Spread pasta on the serving tray and serve with the chickpeas gravy on top
11. Sprinkle dried oregano from top

Nutrition:
Carbs: 47.5g
Protein: 14.8g
Fats: 12.4g
Calories: 304Kcal

338. Chickpeas Tomato Garlic Sauce Macaronis

Preparation Time: 30 minutes
Servings: 2

Ingredients

- Macaronis: 1 cup (after cooking
- Chickpeas: 1 cup rinsed and drained
- Cherry tomatoes: 1 cup diced
- Onions: 1 chopped
- Garlic: 2 cloves
- Vinegar: 3 tbsp
- Olive oil: 2 tbsp
- Tabasco: 4-5 dashes
- Salt: as per your taste
- Pepper: as per your taste

- Spring onion greens: 3 tbsp chopped

Directions:
1. Take a pan and heat oil
2. Add onion and sauté for 5 minutes
3. Add tomatoes and whole garlic cloves and sauté for 5 minutes and stir
4. Add in vinegar, Tabasco, and a lot of salt and pepper
5. Cooking Time: macaroni as per packet instructions and add chickpeas near the end and stir
6. Drain the pasta but keep 2 tablespoons of water and add to tomatoes
7. Add the tomato mixture to the blender and blend
8. Add pasta to the serving tray and mix in tomato sauce
9. Top with spring onion

Nutrition:
Carbs: 52g
Protein: 26.9g
Fats: 17.4g
Calories: 312Kcal

339. Chinese Style Pasta

Preparation Time: 30 minutes
Servings: 4

Ingredients

- Pasta: 2 cups (after cooking
- Olive oil: 2 tbsp
- Garlic: 2 cloves minced
- Red onion: 1 small diced
- Bell pepper: 1 cup diced
- Cabbage: 1 cup diced
- Carrot: 1 cup diced
- Soy sauce: 1 tbsp
- Hot sauce: 1 tbsp
- Salt: 1 tsp
- Black pepper: ½ tsp

- Green onions: 2 tbsp

Directions:
1. Cooking Time: pasta as per packet instructions
2. Take a large saucepan and add olive oil and heat on medium flame
3. Include onion and garlic to the pan and Cooking Time: for a minute
4. Now add bell pepper, cabbage, carrot, salt, soy sauce, hot sauce, and pepper and stir for 5 minutes
5. Then add pasta and mix well
6. Then cover and Cooking Time: for 2 minutes on low flame and remove from heat
7. Sprinkle green onion on top and serve

Nutrition:
Carbs: 29.5g
Protein: 5.4g
Fats: 8.05g
Calories: 205Kcal

340. Cold Szechuan Noodles

Preparation Time: 15minutes
Servings: 2

Ingredients

- Wholewheat noodles: 275g pack
- Sugar snap peas: a handful halved
- Toasted sesame seeds: 1 tbsp
- Cucumber: ½ peeled seeded and chopped
- Sesame oil: 1 tsp
- Red pepper: ½ sliced
- Roughly chopped coriander: a small bunch

For the Dressing:
- Soy sauce: 2 tsp
- Vinegar: 2 tbsp
- Ginger: 3cm piece grated
- Garlic: 1/2 clove crushed

- Peanut butter: 1 tbsp smooth
- Chili oil: 1 tbsp

Directions:

1. Cooking Time: noodles as per packet instructions
2. Take a bowl and add cooked noodles and pour some sesame oil
3. Add red pepper, cucumber and sugar snaps and mix well
4. Mix all dressing ingredients well, ladle over the noodles
5. Sprinkle some sesame seeds and coriander

Nutrition:

Carbs: 46.8g

Protein: 13g

Fats: 17.3g

Calories: 408Kcal

341. Creamy Garlic Pasta

Preparation Time: 30 minutes

Servings: 2

Ingredients

- All-purpose flour: 4 tbsp
- Whole wheat pasta: 1 ¼ cup
- Garlic: 8 large cloves
- Grape tomatoes: 3 cups half
- Shallots: 2 medium diced
- Olive oil
- Salt: as per your taste
- Black pepper: as per your taste
- Unsweetened plain almond milk: 2 ½ cup

Directions:

1. Preheat the oven to 204C
2. Add half tomatoes to the baking sheet lined with parchment paper
3. Brush with olive oil and sprinkle salt on top and bake for 20 minutes
4. Cooking Time: pasta as per packet instructions

5. Prepare sauce side by side, take a pan and add 1 tablespoon of olive oil
6. Add shallot and garlic and stir
7. Sprinkle salt and pepper and mix and Cooking Time: for 4 minutes till it softens
8. Add in flour and mix and add almond milk and again add a pinch of salt and pepper
9. Cooking Time: until thicken and add in garlic
10. Blend the sauce to make it creamier and back to the pan to heat up
11. Now add pasta and top with tomatoes and mix
12. Serve immediately when hot

Nutrition:

Carbs: 63.8 g

Protein: 11.8 g

Fats: 8.9 g

Calories: 378 Kcal

342. Fried Green Pasta

Preparation Time: 30 minutes

Servings: 2

Ingredients

- Pasta: 1 cup cooked
- Long-stemmed broccoli: 1 cup
- Kale: 1 cup
- Olive oil: 1 tbsp
- Peas: 1 cup
- Salt: as per your taste
- Smoked paprika: ½ tsp

Directions:

1. Cooking Time: pasta as per packet instructions
2. Take a pan and heat olive oil
3. Take a bowl and add broccoli, peas, salt, paprika and mix well and add to the pan
4. Fry on low heat for 20 minutes and

turn in between

5. Add kale at the last minutes
6. Mix pasta and season

Nutrition:

Carbs: 42.5g

Protein:13.4g

Fats: 10.5g

Calories:227.2Kcal

343. Gazpacho Spaghetti

Preparation Time: 15 minutes

Servings: 2

Ingredients

- Spaghetti : 160g
- Red onion: ½ roughly chopped
- Green pepper: 1 chopped
- Cherry tomatoes:250g
- Tabasco: a good dash
- Garlic: ½ clove
- Vinegar: 1 tbsp
- Basi l a small bunch

Directions:

1. Cooking Time: pasta as per packet instructions
2. In the meanwhile, take a blender and add tomatoes, garlic, onion, and pepper, and blend
3. Add in salt, Tabasco, and vinegar and combine well
4. Add the sauce to the paste
5. Top with basil and serve

Nutrition:

Carbs: 69g

Protein: 12.7g

Fats: 2.3g

Calories: 364sKcal

344. Garlic Vegetable Pasta

Preparation Time: 40 minutes

Servings: 2

Ingredients

- Pasta: 1 cup (after cooking
- Olive oil: 2 tbsp
- Garlic: 2 cloves minced
- Chickpeas: 1 cup can
- Red onion: 1 small diced
- Bell pepper: 1 cup diced
- Tomatoes: 1 cup diced
- Chili powder: 1 tsp
- Cumin: 1 tsp
- Salt: 1 tsp
- Black pepper: ½ tsp
- Garlic whole: 1
- Cashew cream: ½ cup
- Cilantro: 2 tbsp chopped

Directions:

1. Cooking Time: pasta as per packet instructions
2. Roast garlic in the oven by brushing oil for 30 minutes
3. Take a large saucepan and add olive oil and heat on medium flame
4. Include onion and garlic to the pan and Cooking Time: for a minute
5. Now add bell pepper, tomatoes, chickpeas, cumin, salt, pepper, and chili powder and stir
6. Cooking Time: for 10 minutes
7. Stir the spoon and add cooked pasta
8. Slice roasted garlic and add to the pasta and mix in the cream
9. Cover and Cooking Time: for 2 minutes on low flame and remove from heat
10. Sprinkle cilantro on top and serve

Nutrition:
Carbs: 60g
Protein: 15.4g
Fats: 19.6g
Calories: 543Kcal

345. Gochujang Cauliflower Spaghetti

Preparation Time: 45 minutes
Servings: 2

Ingredients

- Spaghetti: 2 cups
- Olive oil: 2 tbsp
- Cauliflower: 2 cups cut in big florets
- Gochujang: 2 tbsp
- Rice vinegar: 1 tbsp
- Sliced red pepper: 1 cup sliced
- Carrot: 2 sliced
- Salt: as per your taste
- Pepper: as per your taste
- Coriander: 1/2 cup chopped

Directions:

1. Cooking Time: spaghetti as per packet instructions
2. Preheat the oven 200C
3. Add cauliflowers to the baking sheet and sprinkle seasoning and brush with olive oil
4. Roast for 25 minutes till it turns golden and soft
5. Remove from oven and brush with gochujang and Cooking Time: in the oven again for 10 minutes
6. Add to the bowl and mix with carrots and red bell pepper
7. Season with salt, coriander, and pepper and pour vinegar from top
8. Spread spaghetti on the serving tray and top with the cauliflower

Nutrition:
Carbs: 52.5g

Protein: 10.9g
Fats: 15.5g
Calories: 404Kcal

346. Kale Chickpeas Pasta

Preparation Time: 30 minutes
Servings: 2

Ingredients

- Pasta: 1 cup cooked
- Chickpeas: 1 cup rinsed and drained well
- Onion: 1 cup finely diced
- Tomato: 2 cups diced
- Lemon juice: 2 tbsp
- Kale: 1 cup
- Olive oil: 2 tbsp
- Tamari: 1 tbsp
- Coriander: 2 tbsp chopped
- Garlic: 1 clove crushed

Directions:

1. Cooking Time: pasta as per packet instructions
2. Add garlic, lemon juice, tamari, and olive oil in a bowl and whisk
3. Take a serving bowl and combine kale, pasta, chickpeas, onion, tomatoes, and the sauce you made
4. Add coriander from the top and serve

Nutrition:
Carbs: 54g
Protein: 14.6g
Fats: 18g
Calories: 442Kcal

347. Lemon Fusilli With Cauli

Preparation Time: 20 minutes
Servings: 2

Ingredients

- Fusilli: 1 cup cooked
- Cauliflower: 1 cup roughly chopped

- Garlic: 2 cloves thinly sliced
- Olive oil: 1 tbsp
- Chili flakes: 1 tsp
- Salt: as per your taste
- Pepper: as per your taste
- Lemon: 1 juice and zest

Directions:

1. Cooking Time: the pasta as per the packet instruction
2. Add cauliflower when the pasta is about to be done
3. Drain but keep one cup of the water
4. Take a large pan and heat oil
5. Add in garlic and Cooking Time: for two minutes
6. Add in chili and Cooking Time: for a minutes
7. Add pasta, lemon juice and zest, salt, pepper, and cauliflower with the pasta water
8. Mix everything well and serve

Nutrition:

Carbs: 21.6g

Protein: 4.85g

Fats: 7.9g

Calories: 172Kcal

348. Lemony Pasta With Kidney Beans

Preparation Time: 30 minutes

Servings: 4

Ingredients

- Pasta: 2 cups (after cooking
- Onion: 1 chopped
- Garlic: 1 ½ tsp minced
- Cumin: 1 tsp
- Frozen corn: 1 cup
- Cayenne pepper: ¼ tsp
- Kidney beans: 1 cup drained and rinsed

- Fresh cilantro: 2 tsp
- Lemon juice: 3 tbsp
- Cooking oil: 2 tbsp
- Salt: as per your taste

Directions:

1. Cooking Time: pasta as per packet instructions
2. Take a saucepan and heat oil in it
3. Add garlic and onion to it and make them tender
4. Add salt, cayenne pepper, and cumin
5. Now add corns and beans and mix well
6. Cover and Cooking Time: for 5 minutes
7. Add in pasta and stir and remove from heat after 5 minutes
8. Pour lemon juice on top
9. Garnish with cilantro and serve

Nutrition:

Carbs: 41.98g

Protein: 9.3g

Fats: 8.4g

Calories: 274Kcal

349. Lentils Soup Savory Spaghetti

Time:45 minutes

Servings: 2

Ingredients

- Spaghetti: 1 cup cooked
- Red lentils: 1 cup
- Potato: 1 cup diced
- Crushed tomatoes: 2 cups
- Onion: 1 diced
- Ginger: 1 tbsp paste
- Garlic: 1 tbsp paste
- Vegetable oil: 2 tbsp
- Water: 4 cups
- Italian herb seasoning: 1 tbsp

- Salt & pepper: as per your taste

Directions:

1. Cooking Time: spaghetti as per packet instructions
2. Take a large saucepan and heat oil on a medium flame
3. Add onion and ginger and garlic paste and sauté for 3-4 minutes
4. Pour water and bring to boil
5. Add lentils, potatoes, and salt and bring to boil
6. Lower the heat to medium and Cooking Time: for 20 minutes with partial cover
7. Now add crushed tomatoes to the lentils along with Italian herb seasoning and pepper
8. Cooking Time: on low flame for 15 minutes
9. Add the mixture to the high-speed blender to make a puree
10. Add in spaghetti pasta and mix well
11. Add salt and pepper to augment the taste

Nutrition:

Carbs: 33.33g
Protein: 13.3g
Fats: 15.1g
Calories: 335.2Kcal

350. Long-Stemmed Broccoli With Spaghetti

Preparation Time: 20 minutes
Servings: 2

Ingredients

- Wholewheat spaghetti: 150g
- Long-stemmed broccoli: 320g roughly chopped
- Garlic: 2 cloves thinly sliced
- Olive oil: 2 tbsp
- Chili flakes: 1 tsp

- Salt: as per your taste
- Pepper: as per your taste
- Lemon: 1 juice and zest

Directions:

1. Cooking Time: the spaghetti as per the packet instruction
2. Add the broccoli when the pasta is about to be done
3. Drain but keep one cup of the water
4. Take a large pan and heat oil
5. Add in garlic and Cooking Time: for two minutes
6. Add in chili and Cooking Time: for a minutes
7. Add pasta, lemon juice and zest, salt, pepper, and broccoli with the pasta water
8. Mix everything well and serve

Nutrition:

Carbs: 32.6g
Protein: 24.7g
Fats: 28.3g
Calories: 498Kcal

351. Pasta With Beans

Preparation Time: 30 minutes
Servings: 2

Ingredients

- Pasta: 1 cup (after cooking
- Olive oil: 1 tbsp
- Beans: 1 cup can rinsed and drained
- Garlic: 2 cloves minced
- Tomato paste: ¼ cup
- Red onion: 1 small diced
- Red chili flakes: 1 tsp
- Salt: 1 tsp
- Black pepper: ½ tsp
- Parsley: ½ cup

Directions:

1. Cooking Time: pasta as per packet

instructions

2. Take a saucepan and heat oil in it
3. Add minced garlic and onion to it and make them tender
4. Add beans, salt, pepper, tomato paste, and red chili flakes and mix well
5. Add cooked pasta and stir
6. Lower the heat and cover and Cooking Time: for 5 minutes and then remove from heat
7. Sprinkle parsley on top and serve

Nutrition:

Carbs: 39.2g

Protein: 11.3g

Fats: 8.2g

Calories: 272Kcal

352. Peas Tomatoes Macaroni

Preparation Time: 40 minutes

Servings: 2

Ingredients

- Macaroni: 1 cup (after cooking
- Frozen peas: 1 cup rinsed and drained
- Cherry tomatoes: 1 cup diced
- Onions: 1 chopped
- Garlic: 2 cloves
- Vinegar: 3 tbsp
- Olive oil: 2 tbsp
- Tahini: 2 tbsp
- Salt: as per your taste
- Pepper: as per your taste
- Spring onion greens: 3 tbsp chopped

Directions:

1. Take a pan and heat oil
2. Add onion and sauté for 5 minutes
3. Add tomatoes and whole garlic cloves and sauté for 5 minutes and stir
4. Add in vinegar, tahini, and a lot of salt and pepper
5. Cooking Time: macaroni as per packet instructions and add peas at the end
6. Drain the pasta but keep 2 tablespoons of water and add to tomatoes
7. Add the tomato mixture to the blender and blend
8. Combine pasta and tomato mixture
9. Serve with spring onions on top

Nutrition:

Carbs: 37.5g

Protein: 8.9g

Fats: 15.4g

Calories: 320Kcal

353. Penne Bean Pasta With Roasted Tomato Sauce

Preparation Time: 15 minutes

Servings: 2

Ingredients

- Penne: 1 cup (after cooking
- Beans: 1 cup washed and drained
- Cherry tomatoes: 1 cup halved
- Spring onions: 3 chopped
- Vinegar: 3 tbsp
- Olive oil: 3 tbsp
- Tabasco: 4-5 dashes
- Salt: as per your taste
- Pepper: as per your taste
- Basil: 2 tbsp torn

Directions:

1. Roast tomatoes in the oven for 8 minutes
2. Take a bowl and add in roasted tomatoes, olive oil, vinegar, Tabasco, spring onion, and a lot of salt and pepper and mix well
3. Cooking Time: penne as per packet instructions and add bean when it is about to be cooked
4. Drain the pasta but keep 2 tablespoons of water and add to the

sauce

5. Add pasta to the sauce
6. Top with torn basil and serve

Nutrition:
Carbs: 49.9g
Protein: 13.9g
Fats: 22.7g
Calories: 490Kcal

354. Protein-Rich Chickpeas Pasta

Preparation Time: 30 minutes
Servings: 2

Ingredients

- Pasta: 1 cup
- Olive oil: 1 tbsp
- Chickpeas: 1 cup can
- Garlic: 2 cloves minced
- Garlic: 1 tbsp minced
- Red onion: 1 small diced
- Cumin: 1 tsp
- Salt: 1 tsp
- Pepper: ½ tsp
- Hummus: ½ cup

Directions:

1. Cooking Time: pasta as per packet instructions
2. Take a large saucepan and add olive oil and heat on medium flame
3. Include onion, ginger, and garlic to the pan and Cooking Time: for 2-4 minutes
4. Now add chickpeas, cumin, salt, and pepper
5. Stir the spoon and add pasta
6. Lower the heat and cover and Cooking Time: for 2 minutes and mix in hummus and serve

Nutrition:
Carbs: 61.8g
Protein: 18.9g

Fats: 18.9g
Calories: 488Kcal

355. Protein-Rich Zucchini Pasta

Preparation Time: 30 minutes
Servings: 2

Ingredients

- Pasta: 1 cup (after cooked
- Olive oil: 1 tbsp
- Vegetable broth: ½ cup
- Black beans: 1 cup
- Garlic: 2 cloves minced
- Zucchini: 1 cup diced
- Red onion: 1 small diced
- Chili powder: 1 tsp
- Cumin: 1 tsp
- Salt: 1 tsp
- Black pepper: ½ tsp
- Fresh cilantro: 2 tbsp

Directions:

1. Take a large saucepan and add olive oil and heat on medium flame
2. Include onion and garlic to the pan and Cooking Time: for a minute
3. Now add zucchini, black beans, cumin, salt, chili powder, and broth
4. Stir the spoon and let them boil
5. Lower the heat and cover and Cooking Time: for 10 minutes
6. In the meanwhile, Cooking Time: pasta as per packet instructions
7. When done, add to the beans
8. Sprinkle salt, pepper, and cilantro on top and serve

Nutrition:
Carbs: 28.15g
Protein: 12.35g
Fats: 8.5g
Calories: 287Kcal

356. Raw Garlic Tomato Sauce Spaghetti

Preparation Time: 15 minutes
Servings: 2

Ingredients

- Spaghetti: 1 cup (after cooking
- Cherry tomatoes: 4 halved
- Spring onions: 3 chopped
- Garlic: 3 cloves minced
- Vinegar: 3 tbsp
- Olive oil: 2 tbsp
- Tabasco: 5 dashes
- Salt: as per your taste
- Pepper: as per your taste
- Basil: 2 tbsp torn

Directions:

1. Take a bowl and add in cherry tomatoes, minced garlic, olive oil, vinegar, Tabasco, spring onion, and a lot of salt and pepper
2. Cooking Time: spaghetti as per packet instructions
3. Drain the pasta but keep 2 tablespoons of water and add to the sauce
4. Blend the sauce by removing tomatoes
5. Add pasta to the sauce and mix in tomatoes
6. Top with basil and serve

Nutrition:
Carbs: 21.8g
Protein: 8.45g
Fats: 15.95g
Calories: 379Kcal

357. Red Pesto Pasta

Preparation Time: 10 minutes
Servings: 4

Ingredients

- Pasta: 4 cups cooked
- Red cabbage: 1 head small
- Garlic: 2 cloves
- Lemon juice: 3 tbsp
- Pepper: ½ tsp
- Ground almonds: 2 tbsp
- Extra-virgin olive oil: 3 tbsp
- Salt: as per your need
- Chili sauce: 1 tbsp

Directions:

1. Prepare pasta as per packet instructions
2. Roast cabbage in the oven for 10 minutes at 160C
3. Take a blender and add all the ingredients including roasted cabbage
4. Blend them well
5. Mix pasta to the paste and season with more salt and pepper

Nutrition:
Carbs: 31.8g
Protein: 13.8g
Fats: 35.2g
Calories: 468Kcal

358. Roasted Broccoli With Pasta

Preparation Time: 30 minutes
Servings: 2

Ingredients

- Pasta: 1 cup (after cooking
- Broccoli florets: 1 cup
- Olive oil: 1 tbsp
- Cashew cream: ½ cup
- Green onion: 1 chopped

- Salt and pepper: as per your taste

Directions:
1. Cooking Time: pasta as per packet instructions
2. Preheat the oven to 400F
3. In a bowl, add broccoli and season with pepper and salt and brush with oil
4. Add them to the baking sheet and roast for 20 minutes
5. In a serving tray, spread pasta and top with roasted broccoli
6. Spread cashew cream on top
7. Sprinkle green onions on top and serve

Nutrition:
Carbs: 26.2g
Protein: 6.7g
Fats: 9.65g
Calories: 204Kcal

359. Roasted Veggie Lemon Salad

Preparation Time: 30 minutes
Servings: 4

Ingredients
- Macaroni pasta: 4 cups
- Carrots: 1 cup sliced
- Broccoli: 1 cup sliced
- Cauliflower: 1 cup sliced
- Olive oil: 1 tbsp
- Salt: as per your taste
- Pepper: as per your taste

For the Dressing:
- Lemon: 2 zest and juice
- Mustard: 1 tbsp
- Vinegar: 2 tsp
- Garlic: 1 clove crushed
- Extra-virgin olive oil: 2 tbsp
- Salt: as per your need

Directions:
1. Cooking Time: pasta as per packet instructions
2. Add all the vegetables to the baking tray, sprinkle salt and pepper, brush with olive oil and bake for 20 minutes
3. Prepare the dressing by adding all the ingredients except oil and combine it slowly at the end whisking to gain the correct consistency
4. Add pasta to the tray, and spread vegetables to the tray and pour dressing from the top and serve

Nutrition:
Carbs: 41.5g
Protein: 10.7g
Fats: 8.1g
Calories: 399Kcal

360. Savory Chickpeas Pasta

Preparation Time: 40 minutes
Servings: 2

Ingredients
- Pasta: 1 cup cooked
- Chickpeas: 1 cup
- Vegetable broth: 2 cups
- Olive oil: 1 tbsp
- Garlic: 2 cloves minced
- Red bell pepper: ½ cup chopped
- Onion: 1 medium minced
- Tomatoes: 1 cup chopped
- Black pepper: ¼ tsp
- Carrot: 1 diced
- Dried parsley: ½ tsp
- Tomato paste: 1 tbsp
- Salt: as per your need

Directions:
1. Cooking Time: pasta as per packet instructions
2. Cooking Time: chickpeas by soaking

them overnight and boiling them for two hours on medium heat

3. Take a large saucepan and heat oil on medium flame
4. Add onions and Cooking Time: for 3-4 minutes
5. Add garlic and Cooking Time: for a minute and stir
6. Add tomatoes, bell pepper, carrot, chickpeas, oregano, tomato sauce, and parsley
7. Stir for around a minute or two
8. Add vegetable broth, cover, and boil
9. Simmer for 20-25 minutes until thickened
10. To give a better texture, mash some chickpeas with the back of the spoon
11. Add pasta to the chickpeas soup
12. Season with salt, and pepper

Nutrition:
Carbs: 56.4g
Protein: 14.47g
Fats: 17.7g
Calories: 442Kcal

361. Saucy Brussels Macaroni

Preparation Time: 30 minutes
Servings: 2

Ingredients
- Macaroni: 1 cup (after cooking
- Brussels sprout: 1 cup halved
- Olive oil: 1 tbsp
- Almond milk: ½ cup
- Flour: 2 tbsp
- Green onion: 1 chopped
- Salt and pepper: as per your taste
- Dried oregano: 2 tbsp

Directions:
1. Cooking Time: pasta as per packet instructions
2. Preheat the oven to 400F

3. In a bowl, add Brussels sprouts and season with pepper and salt and brush with oil
4. Add them to the baking sheet and roast for 20 minutes
5. In a serving tray, spread pasta and top with roasted sprouts
6. In a small pan, heat almond milk and stir in flour
7. Add pasta and sprouts to them and stir to thicken
8. Serve with oregano on top

Nutrition:
Carbs: 49.75g
Protein: 6.75g
Fats: 9.65g
Calories: 204Kcal

SAUCES, AND CONDIMENTS

362. Green Goddess Hummus

Preparation time: 5 minutes
Cooking time: 0 minute
Servings: 6
Ingredients:

- ¼ cup tahini
- ¼ cup lemon juice
- 2 tablespoons olive oil
- ½ cup chopped parsley
- ¼ cup chopped basil
- 3 tablespoons chopped chives
- 1 large clove of garlic, peeled, chopped
- ½ teaspoon salt
- 15-ounce cooked chickpeas
- 2 tablespoons water

Directions:

1. Place all the ingredients in the order in a food processor or blender and then pulse for 3 to 5 minutes at high speed until the thick mixture comes together.
2. Tip the hummus in a bowl and then serve.

Nutrition Value:
Calories: 110.4 Cal
Fat: 6 g
Carbs: 11.5 g
Protein: 4.8 g
Fiber: 2.6 g

363. Garlic, Parmesan And White Bean Hummus

Preparation time: 5 minutes
Cooking time: 0 minute
Servings: 6
Ingredients:

- 4 cloves of garlic, peeled
- 12 ounces cooked white beans
- 1/8 teaspoon salt
- ½ lemon, zested
- 1 tablespoon lemon juice
- 1 tablespoon olive oil
- 3 tablespoon water
- 1/4 cup grated Parmesan cheese

Directions:

1. Place all the ingredients in the order in a food processor or blender and then pulse for 3 to 5 minutes at high speed until the thick mixture comes together.
2. Tip the hummus in a bowl and then serve.

Nutrition Value:
Calories: 90 Cal
Fat: 7 g
Carbs: 5 g
Protein: 2 g
Fiber: 1 g

364. Tomato Jam

Preparation time: 10 minutes
Cooking time: 20 minutes
Servings: 16
Ingredients:

- 2 pounds tomatoes
- ¼ teaspoon. ground black pepper
- ½ teaspoon. salt
- ¼ cup coconut sugar
- ½ teaspoon. white wine vinegar
- ¼ teaspoon. smoked paprika

Directions:
1. Place a large pot filled with water over medium heat, bring it to boil, then add tomatoes and boil for 1 minute.
2. Transfer tomatoes to a bowl containing chilled water, let them stand for 2 minutes, and then peel them by hand.
3. Cut the tomatoes, remove and discard seeds, then chop tomatoes and place them in a large pot.
4. Sprinkle sugar over coconut, stir until mixed and let it stand for 10 minutes.
5. Then place the pot over medium-high heat, Cooking Time: for 15 minutes, then add remaining ingredients except for vinegar and Cooking Time: for 10 minutes until thickened.
6. Remove pot from heat, stir in vinegar and serve.

Nutrition Value:
Calories: 17.6 Cal
Fat: 1.3 g
Carbs: 1.5 g
Protein: 0.2 g
Fiber: 0.3 g

365. Kale And Walnut Pesto

Preparation time: 5 minutes
Cooking time: 10 minutes
Servings: 4
Ingredients:
- 1/2 bunch kale, leaves chop
- 1/2 cup chopped walnuts
- 2 cloves of garlic, peeled
- 1/4 cup nutritional yeast
- ½ of lemon, juiced
- 1/4 cup olive oil
- ¼ teaspoon. ground black pepper
- 1/3 teaspoon. salt

Directions:

1. Place a large pot filled with water over medium heat, bring it to boil, then add kale and boil for 5 minutes until tender.
2. Drain kale, then transfer it in a blender, add remaining ingredients and then pulse for 5 minutes until smooth.
3. Serve straight away.

Nutrition Value:
Calories: 344 Cal
Fat: 29 g
Carbs: 16 g
Protein: 9 g
Fiber: 6 g

366. Buffalo Chicken Dip

Preparation time: 5 minutes
Cooking time: 15 minutes
Servings: 4
Ingredients:
- 2 cups cashews
- 2 teaspoons garlic powder
- 1 1/2 teaspoons salt
- 2 teaspoons onion powder
- 3 tablespoons lemon juice
- 1 cup buffalo sauce
- 1 cup of water
- 14-ounce artichoke hearts, packed in water, drained

Directions:
1. Switch on the oven, then set it to 375 degrees F and let it preheat.
2. Meanwhile, pour 3 cups of boiling water in a bowl, add cashews and let soak for 5 minutes.
3. Then drain the cashew, transfer them into the blender, pour in water, add lemon juice and all the seasoning and blend until smooth.
4. Add artichokes and buffalo sauce,

process until chunky mixture comes together, and then transfer the dip to an ovenproof dish.

5. Bake for 20 minutes and then serve.

Nutrition Value:

Calories: 100 Cal

Fat: 100 g

Carbs: 100 g

Protein: 100 g

Fiber: 100 g

367. Barbecue Tahini Sauce

Preparation time: 5 minutes

Cooking time: 0 minute

Servings: 8

Ingredients:

- 6 tablespoons tahini
- 3/4 teaspoon garlic powder
- 1/8 teaspoon red chili powder
- 2 teaspoons maple syrup
- 1/4 teaspoon salt
- 3 teaspoons molasses
- 3 teaspoons apple cider vinegar
- 1/4 teaspoon liquid smoke
- 10 teaspoons tomato paste
- 1/2 cup water

Directions:

1. Place all the ingredients in the order in a food processor or blender and then pulse for 3 to 5 minutes at high speed until smooth.
2. Tip the sauce in a bowl and then serve.

Nutrition Value:

Calories: 86 Cal

Fat: 5 g

Carbs: 7 g

Protein: 2 g

Fiber: 0 g

368. Vegan Ranch Dressing

Preparation time: 5 minutes

Cooking time: 0 minute

Servings: 16

Ingredients:

- 1/4 teaspoon. ground black pepper
- 2 teaspoon. chopped parsley
- 1/2 teaspoon. garlic powder
- 1 tablespoon chopped dill
- 1/2 teaspoon. onion powder
- 1 cup vegan mayonnaise
- 1/2 cup soy milk, unsweetened

Directions:

1. Take a medium bowl, add all the ingredients in it and then whisk until combined.
2. Serve straight away

Nutrition Value:

Calories: 16 Cal

Fat: 9 g

Carbs: 0 g

Protein: 0 g

Fiber: 0 g

369. Cashew Yogurt

Preparation time: 12 hours and 5 minutes

Cooking time: 0 minute

Servings: 8

Ingredients:

- 3 probiotic supplements
- 2 2/3 cups cashews, unsalted , soaked in warm water for 15 minutes
- 1/4 teaspoon sea salt
- 4 tablespoon lemon juice
- 1 1/2 cup water

Directions:

1. Drain the cashews, add them into the food processor, then add remaining ingredients, except for probiotic supplements, and pulse for 2 minutes

until smooth.

2. Tip the mixture in a bowl, add probiotic supplements, stir until mixed, then cover the bowl with a cheesecloth and let it stand for 12 hours in a dark and cool room.

3. Serve straight away.

Nutrition Value:

Calories: 252 Cal

Fat: 19.8 g

Carbs: 14.1 g

Protein: 8.3 g

Fiber: 1.5 g

370. Nacho Cheese Sauce

Preparation time: 15 minutes

Cooking time: 5 minutes

Servings: 12

Ingredients:

- 2 cups cashews, unsalted , soaked in warm water for 15 minutes
- 2 teaspoons salt
- 1/2 cup nutritional yeast
- 1 teaspoon garlic powder
- 1/2 teaspoon smoked paprika
- 1/2 teaspoon red chili powder
- 1 teaspoon onion powder
- 2 teaspoons Sriracha
- 3 tablespoons lemon juice
- 4 cups water, divided

Directions:

1. Drain the cashews, transfer them to a food processor, then add remaining ingredients, reserving 3 cups water, and , and pulse for 3 minutes until smooth.

2. Tip the mixture in a saucepan, place it over medium heat and Cooking Time: for 3 to 5 minutes until the sauce has thickened and bubbling, whisking constantly.

3. When done, taste the sauce to adjust seasoning and then serve.

Nutrition Value:

Calories: 128 Cal

Fat: 10 g

Carbs: 8 g

Protein: 5 g

Fiber: 1 g

371. Thai Peanut Sauce

Preparation time: 10 minutes

Cooking time: 10 minutes

Servings: 4

Ingredients:

- 2 tablespoons ground peanut, and more for topping
- 2 tablespoons Thai red curry paste
- ½ teaspoon salt
- 1 tablespoon sugar
- 1/2 cup creamy peanut butter
- 2 tablespoons apple cider vinegar
- 3/4 cup coconut milk, unsweetened

Directions:

1. Take a saucepan, place it over low heat, add all the ingredients, whisk well until combined, and then bring the sauce to simmer.

2. Then remove the pan from heat, top with ground peanuts, and serve.

Nutrition Value:

Calories: 397 Cal

Fat: 50 g

Carbs: 16 g

Protein: 26 g

Fiber: 4 g

372. Garlic Alfredo Sauce

Preparation time: 10 minutes

Cooking time: 5 minutes

Servings: 4

Ingredients:

- 1 1/2 cups cashews, unsalted , soaked in warm water for 15 minutes
- 6 cloves of garlic, peeled, minced
- 1/2 medium sweet onion, peeled, chopped
- 1 teaspoon salt
- 1/4 cup nutritional yeast
- 1 tablespoon lemon juice
- 2 tablespoons olive oil
- 2 cups almond milk, unsweetened
- 12 ounces fettuccine pasta, cooked, for serving

Directions:

1. Take a small saucepan, place it over medium heat, add oil and when hot, add onion and garlic, and Cooking Time: for 5 minutes until sauté.
2. Meanwhile, drain the cashews, transfer them into a food processor, add remaining ingredients including onion mixture, except for pasta, and pulse for 3 minutes until very smooth.
3. Pour the prepared sauce over pasta, toss until coated and serve.

Nutrition Value:
Calories: 439 Cal
Fat: 20 g
Carbs: 52 g
Protein: 15 g
Fiber: 4 g

373. Spicy Red Wine Tomato Sauce

Preparation time: 5 minutes
Cooking time: 1 hour
Servings: 4
Ingredients:

- 28 ounces puree of whole tomatoes, peeled
- 4 cloves of garlic, peeled
- 1 tablespoon dried basil

- ¼ teaspoon ground black pepper
- 1 tablespoon dried oregano
- ¼ teaspoon red pepper flakes
- 1 tablespoon dried sage
- 1 tablespoon dried thyme
- 3 teaspoon coconut sugar
- 1/2 of lemon, juice
- 1/4 cup red wine

Directions:

1. Take a large saucepan, place it over medium heat, add tomatoes and remaining ingredients, stir and simmer for 1 hour or more until thickened and cooked.
2. Serve sauce over pasta.

Nutrition Value:
Calories: 110 Cal
Fat: 2.5 g
Carbs: 9 g
Protein: 2 g
Fiber: 2 g

374. Vodka Cream Sauce

Preparation time: 5 minutes
Cooking time: 5 minutes
Servings: 1
Ingredients:

- 1/4 cup cashews, unsalted , soaked in warm water for 15 minutes
- 24-ounce marinara sauce
- 2 tablespoons vodka
- 1/4 cup water

Directions:

1. Drain the cashews, transfer them in a food processor, pour in water, and blend for 2 minutes until smooth.
2. Tip the mixture in a pot, stir in pasta sauce and vodka and simmer for 3 minutes over medium heat until done, stirring constantly.
3. Serve sauce over pasta.

Nutrition Value:
Calories: 207 Cal
Fat: 16 g
Carbs: 9.2 g
Protein: 2.4 g
Fiber: 4.3 g

375. Hot Sauce

Preparation time: 10 minutes
Cooking time: 15 minutes
Servings: 6
Ingredients:

- 4 Serrano peppers, destemmed
- 1/2 of medium white onion, chopped
- 1 medium carrot, chopped
- 10 habanero chilies, destemmed
- 6 cloves of garlic, unpeeled
- 2 teaspoons sea salt
- 1 cup apple cider vinegar
- 1/2 teaspoon brown rice syrup
- 1 cup of water

Directions:

1. Take a skillet pan, place it medium heat, add garlic, and Cooking Time: for 15 minutes until roasted, frequently turning garlic, set aside to cool.
2. Meanwhile, take a saucepan, place it over medium-low heat, add remaining ingredients in it, except for salt and syrup, stir and Cooking Time: for 12 minutes until vegetables are tender.
3. When the garlic has roasted and cooled, peel them and add them to a food processor.
4. Then add cooked saucepan along with remaining ingredients, and pulse for 3 minutes until smooth.
5. Let sauce cool and then serve straight away

Nutrition Value:
Calories: 137 Cal
Fat: 0 g
Carbs: 30 g
Protein: 4 g
Fiber: 10 g

376. Hot Sauce

Preparation time: 5 minutes
Cooking time: 0 minute
Servings: 16
Ingredients:

- 4 cloves of garlic, peeled
- 15 Hot peppers, de-stemmed, chopped
- 1/2 teaspoon. coriander
- 1/2 teaspoon. sea salt
- 1/2 teaspoon. red chili powder
- 1/2 of lime, zested
- 1/4 teaspoon. cumin
- 1/2 lime, juiced
- 1 cup apple cider vinegar

Directions:

1. Place all the ingredients in the order in a food processor or blender and then pulse for 3 to 5 minutes at high speed until smooth.
2. Tip the sauce in a bowl and then serve.

Nutrition Value:
Calories: 5 Cal
Fat: 0 g
Carbs: 1 g
Protein: 0 g
Fiber: 0.3 g

377. Barbecue Sauce

Preparation time: 5 minutes
Cooking time: 0 minute
Servings: 16
Ingredients:

- 8 ounces tomato sauce
- 1 teaspoon garlic powder
- ¼ teaspoon ground black pepper
- 1/2 teaspoon. sea salt
- 2 Tablespoons Dijon mustard
- 3 packets stevia
- 1 teaspoon molasses
- 1 Tablespoon apple cider vinegar
- 2 Tablespoons tamari
- 1 teaspoon liquid aminos

Directions:

1. Take a medium bowl, place all the ingredients in it, and stir until combined.
2. Serve straight away

Nutrition Value:
Calories: 29 Cal
Fat: 0.1 g
Carbs: 7 g
Protein: 0.1 g
Fiber: 0.1 g

378. Bolognese Sauce

Preparation time: 10 minutes
Cooking time: 45 minutes
Servings: 8
Ingredients:

- ½ of small green bell pepper, chopped
- 1 stalk of celery, chopped
- 1 small carrot, chopped
- 1 medium white onion, peeled, chopped
- 2 teaspoons minced garlic
- 1/2 teaspoon crushed red pepper flakes
- 3 tablespoons olive oil
- 8-ounce tempeh, crumbled
- 8 ounces white mushrooms, chopped
- 1/2 cup dried red lentils
- 28-ounce crushed tomatoes
- 28-ounce whole tomatoes, chopped
- 1 teaspoon dried oregano
- 1/2 teaspoon fennel seed
- 1/2 teaspoon ground black pepper
- 1/2 teaspoon salt
- 1 teaspoon dried basil
- 1/4 cup chopped parsley
- 1 bay leaf
- 6-ounce tomato paste
- 1 cup dry red wine

Directions:

1. Take a Dutch oven, place it over medium heat, add oil, and when hot, add the first six ingredients, stir and Cooking Time: for 5 minutes until sauté.
2. Then switch heat to medium-high level, add two ingredients after olive oil, stir and Cooking Time: for 3 minutes.
3. Switch heat to medium-low level, stir in tomato paste, and continue cooking for 2 minutes.
4. Add remaining ingredients except for lentils, stir and bring the mixture to boil.
5. Switch heat to the low level, simmer sauce for 10 minutes, covering the pan partially, then add lentils and continue cooking for 20 minutes until tender.
6. Serve sauce with cooked pasta.

Nutrition Value:
Calories: 208.8 Cal
Fat: 12 g
Carbs: 17.8 g
Protein: 10.6 g
Fiber: 3.8 g

379. Alfredo Sauce

Preparation time: 5 minutes
Cooking time: 0 minute
Servings: 4
Ingredients:

- 1 cup cashews, unsalted, soaked in warm water for 15 minutes
- 1 teaspoon minced garlic
- 1/4 teaspoon ground black pepper
- 1/3 teaspoon salt
- 1/4 cup nutritional yeast
- 2 tablespoons tamari
- 2 tablespoons olive oil
- 4 tablespoons water

Directions:

1. Drain the cashews, transfer them into a food processor, add remaining ingredients in it, and pulse for 3 minutes until thick sauce comes together.
2. Serve straight away.

Nutrition Value:
Calories: 105.7 Cal
Fat: 5.3 g
Carbs: 11 g
Protein: 4.7 g
Fiber: 2 g

380. Garden Pesto

Preparation time: 5 minutes
Cooking time: 0 minute
Servings: 10
Ingredients:

- 1/4 cup pistachios, shelled

- 3/4 cup parsley leaves
- 1 cup cilantro leaves
- ½ teaspoon minced garlic
- 1/4 cup mint leaves
- 1 cup basil leaves
- ¼ teaspoon ground black pepper
- 1/3 teaspoon salt
- 1/2 cup olive oil
- 1 1/2 teaspoons miso
- 2 teaspoons lemon juice

Directions:

1. Place all the ingredients in the order in a food processor or blender and then pulse for 3 to 5 minutes at high speed until smooth.
2. Tip the pesto in a bowl and then serve.

Nutrition Value:
Calories: 111.5 Cal
Fat: 11.5 g
Carbs: 2.8 g
Protein: 1.2 g
Fiber: 1.4 g

381. Cilantro And Parsley Hot Sauce

Preparation time: 5 minutes
Cooking time: 0 minute
Servings: 4
Ingredients:

- 2 cups of parsley and cilantro leaves with stems
- 4 Thai bird chilies, destemmed, deseeded, torn
- 2 teaspoons minced garlic
- 1 teaspoon salt
- 1/4 teaspoon coriander seed, ground
- 1/4 teaspoon ground black pepper
- 1/2 teaspoon cumin seeds, ground
- 3 green cardamom pods, toasted,

ground

- 1/2 cup olive oil

Directions:

1. Take a spice blender or a food processor, place all the ingredients in it, and process for 5 minutes until the smooth paste comes together.
2. Serve straight away.

Nutrition Value:

Calories: 130 Cal

Fat: 14 g

Carbs: 2 g

Protein: 1 g

Fiber: 1 g

382. Potato Carrot Gravy

Preparation Time: 20 Minutes

Servings: 2 cups of gravy

Ingredients:

- 1 potato, peeled and chopped
- ½ lb (about 4carrots, chopped
- 2 cups water
- 1 tsp garlic powder
- 1 tsp onion powder
- 1 tsp salt
- 1/2 tsp turmeric
- 2 tbsp nutritional yeast
- 2 tsp soy sauce

Directions:

1. Add potato and carrot to Instant Pot along with water.
2. Cover the pot with lid. Set steam release handle to 'sealing' and switch on manual button for 7 minutes over high-pressure.
3. When the timer beeps, allow it to naturally release steam for 5 minutes and then change stem handle to 'venting' to release any remaining steam.
4. Add in rest of the ingredients to

Instant Pot® and using an immersion blender, make gravy directly in Instant Pot.
5. To make the gravy thinner just add a bit more water.

383. Instant Pot Sriracha Sauce

Preparation Time: 30 Minutes

Servings: 2 cups of Sriracha

Ingredients:

- 1 lb red chili peppers (jalapeno, Fresno, etc.
- 6 garlic cloves, peeled
- ½ cup distilled vinegar
- 3 tbsp brown sugar
- 1/3 cup water
- 1 tbsp salt

Directions:

1. Chop chili peppers and put them into a blender.
2. Add remaining ingredients into the blender and blend over high until smooth.
3. Pour this mixture into Instant Pot. Switch on sautée button. Then set 'Adjust' button two times to change heat setting to 'Less'.
4. Let the mixture sauté for about 15 minutes stirring occasionally. After 15 minutes, allow the sauce to cool for about 15 minutes.
5. Store the sriracha in glass containers and keep it in the fridge for 2 weeks.

384. Healthy One-Pot Hummus

Preparation Time: 1 HR 15 Minutes

Servings: 2

Ingredients:

- 1 cup dry garbanzo beans
- 2 cups water
- ½ tsp salt
- 1 tsp cumin

- 2 garlic cloves
- Juice of ½ lemon

Directions:

1. Rinse and drain garbanzo beans. Add beans and water to Instant Pot and Cooking Time: for 1 hour over manual setting, high pressure. Set steam release handle to 'sealing'.
2. When the timer beeps, using quick release Directions, release the steam immediately.
3. Place garbanzo beans along with remaining ingredients in a blender. Use the reserved water after cooking beans.
4. Blend the mixture over high until creamy smooth and serve.

385. Mushroom Gravy

Preparation Time: 20 Minutes
Servings: 10
Ingredients:

- 2 cups sliced fresh mushrooms
- 1½ cups plus 2 tablespoons vegetable or mushroom broth
- 2 tablespoons dry red or white wine
- ¼ cup minced yellow onion
- ½ teaspoon ground dried thyme
- ¼ teaspoon ground sage
- Salt and freshly ground black pepper
- ½ to 1 teaspoon vegan gravy browner

Directions:

1. Combine the onion and 2 tablespoons of broth in the open instant pot on low and simmer until the onion softens.
2. Add the mushrooms and soften more before adding the sage, thyme, and wine.
3. Add half the broth and boil.
4. Reduce the heat and simmer 5

minutes.
5. Add the remaining broth, then put into a blender and make smooth.
6. Put back into the instant pot, salt and pepper, then seal and Cooking Time: on Stew for 10 minutes.
7. Depressurize naturally and serve hot.

386. Creamy Cheesy Sauce

Preparation Time: 6 Minutes
Servings: 2 cups
Ingredients:

- 1cup cashews, soaked
- ½teaspoon vegetable broth powder
- 1teaspoon Dijon mustard
- ½teaspoon paprika
- ½teaspoon garlic powder
- 2tablespoons fresh lemon juice
- ½teaspoon salt
- ½cup nutritional yeast
- 1cup almond milk
- ½teaspoon onion powder

Directions:

1. Add the cashews in a blender.
2. Add the mustard, lemon juice, yeast, onion, salt, garlic, paprika, broth powder and blend into a smooth paste.
3. Serve with curry.

387. Homemade Cashew Cream Cheese

Preparation Time: 15 Minutes
Servings: 2 cups
Ingredients:

- 1cup raw cashews, soaked for 4 hours
- 1teaspoon white miso paste
- 1tablespoon apple cider vinegar
- ½teaspoon salt
- 1teaspoon agave nectar

- 6ounces firm silken tofu
- 2tablespoons fresh lemon juice

Directions:

1. Drain the cashew and add to a blender.
2. Add the agave, salt, miso, vinegar and lemon juice.
3. Blend again into a smooth paste.
4. Add the tofu and blend again.
5. Store in the fridge.

388. Sunflower Seed, Potato & Brown Lentil Pâté

Preparation Time: 15 Minutes
Servings: 6-8
Ingredients:

- 1cup unsalted sunflower seeds, soaked overnight
- ½cup nutritional yeast
- 1onion, chopped
- 1potato, peeled and chopped
- 1½cups brown lentils, cooked
- ⅓cup whole-grain flour
- ¾cup walnut pieces
- 2tablespoons vital wheat gluten
- 1tablespoon olive oil
- 1teaspoon dried thyme
- 3garlic cloves, chopped
- 2tablespoons soy sauce
- ½teaspoon black pepper
- 1teaspoon sweet paprika
- 1teaspoon salt
- 2tablespoons chopped parsley
- ⅛teaspoon ground allspice
- ½teaspoon ground sage
- ⅛teaspoon cayenne pepper

Directions:

1. In an instant pot toss the garlic, onion with some water for 1 minute.
2. Drain the lentils and sunflower seeds.
3. Add the walnuts and sunflower seeds in a blender.
4. Blend into a smooth mix and add the onion mix.
5. Add the lentils, potato and blend again.
6. Add the rest of the ingredients one by one.
7. Blend well to make a smooth paste.
8. Add the mixture to a baking pan.
9. Cover the top using aluminum foil. Make some holes on top.
10. Add to the instant pot and Cooking Time: for 8 minutes.
11. Serve at room temperature.

389. Chickpea & Artichoke Mushroom Pâté

Preparation Time: 15 Minutes
Servings: 6-8
Ingredients:

- 2cups canned artichoke hearts, drained
- 1½cups cooked chickpeas
- 3garlic cloves, chopped
- 1tablespoon fresh lemon juice
- 1 teaspoon dried basil
- ½cup raw cashews, soaked overnight and drained
- 1cup chopped mushrooms
- Shredded fresh basil leaves, for garnish
- 1cup crumbled extra-firm tofu
- Salt and black pepper
- Paprika, for garnish

Directions:

1. In an instant pot add some oil and toss the garlic, mushroom and artichokes for 1 minute.
2. Drain them to get rid of excess liquid.

3. Add the cashews, tofu in a blender and blend until smooth.
4. Add the artichoke mixture, lemon juice, salt, chickpeas, basil and pepper.
5. Blend again and pour into a loaf pan.
6. Cover with aluminum foil and poke some holes on top.
7. Add to your instant pot and Cooking Time: for about 3 minutes.
8. Let it cool down and refrigerate until served.
9. Garnish using basil, paprika.

390. Vegan Sauce

Preparation Time: 5 Minutes
Servings: 1 ¾ cups
Ingredients:
- 2tablespoons yeast extract
- 2tablespoons salt
- 1½cups vegetarian broth
- 2tablespoons vegan gravy browner

Directions:
1. Combine the yeast, vegetarian broth and salt in a bowl.
2. Mix well and add the gravy browner.
3. Mix well and store in a container.

391. Pumpkin Butter

Preparation Time: 30 Minutes
 Servings: 2 Cups
Ingredients:
- 1 15 Ounce Can Pure Pumpkin
- 1 Tablespoon Lemon Juice
- 1/4 Teaspoon Cinnamon
- 1/8 Teaspoon Ground Cloves
- 1/4 Cup Maple Syrup or Agave
- 2/3 Cup Coconut Sugar, muscovado sugar, or maple sugar
- 1 Cup Water- For bottom of instant pot

Directions:
1. Mix pumpkin, lemon juice, cinnamon, cloves, and syrup or agave in an oven-safe bowl.
2. Add coconut sugar or other sugar and cover bowl with foil.
3. Place the steam rack into the instant pot and fill with water.
4. Place the oven safe bowl on the steam rack. On manual setting, Cooking Time: for 25 minutes on high pressure.
5. Quick release or let pressure dissolve on its own.
6. Remove foil and stir. Add more spices if needed.
7. For thicker butter spread, remove steam rack and in the empty instant pot, pour in contents and saute on low setting, stirring occasionally until it thickens.
8. Use as a spread for breads, pancakes, or oatmeal topping. Enjoy!

392. Vegan Cheese Dip

Preparation Time: 30 Mins
Servings: 10
Ingredients:
- 1 7.1 Ounce Daiya Medium Cheddar Style Block or other block vegan cheese, cubed
- 1 8 Ounce Bag Daiya Pepperjack Style Shreds
- 1 Tablespoon Vegan Butter
- 1 Tub Daiya Plain Cream Cheeze Style Spread, Tofu Cream Cheese, or other vegan cream cheese spread
- 1 Tablespoon Garlic Powder
- 1 Teaspoon Turmeric
- 1 Tablespoon Unsweetened Plain Almond Milk
- 1 Tablespoon Dried Oregano

- 1 Cup Water

Directions:
1. Place all ingredients in the instant pot and seal.
2. Use the manual setting and set to 5 minutes.
3. Quick release and remove lid when done cooking.
4. Whisk immediately until smooth. Enjoy!

393. Artichoke Spinach Dip

Preparation Time: 5 Minutes
Servings: 3 ½ cups
Ingredients:
- 1(10-ouncepackage spinach, chopped
- ⅓cup nutritional yeast
- 2(8-ouncejars marinated artichoke hearts
- ½teaspoon Tabasco sauce
- 3scallions, minced
- 1tablespoon fresh lemon juice
- 1cup vegan cream cheese
- ½teaspoon salt

Directions:
1. Drain the artichoke hearts and chop them finely.
2. Add the scallions, lemon juice, salt, artichoke hearts, sauce, spinach and yeast in an instant pot.
3. Cover and Cooking Time: for about 3 minutes.
4. Add the cheese and stir well.
5. Serve warm.

394. Chipotle Bean Cheesy Dip

Preparation Time: 10 Minutes
Servings: 3 cups
Ingredients:
- 2cups pinto beans, cooked, mashed
- 1tablespoon chipotle chiles in adobo, minced
- ¼cup water
- ½cup shredded vegan cheddar cheese
- ¾cup tomato salsa
- 1teaspoon chili powder
- Salt

Directions:
1. In a bowl combine the mashed beans, chipotle chile, salsa, chili powder and water in an instant pot.
2. Mix well and cover with lid.
3. Cooking Time: for about 5 minutes.
4. Add the cheddar cheese and salt and serve warm.
5. Drain the tomatoes and add to a blender.

395. Pasta Sauce From Bologna

Preparation Time: 5 Minutes
Servings: 6
Ingredients:
- 2 tablespoons olive oil
- 2 14oz. can crushed tomatoes
- ¼ cup basil leaves
- ¼ cup chopped parsley
- 1 onion, chopped
- 3 tablespoons lemon juice
- 2 celery stalks, diced
- 2 carrots, grated
- 2 cloves garlic, minced
- Salt and pepper, to taste

Directions:
1. Heat olive oil into Instant pot.
2. Add onion, carrots, and celery. Cooking Time: 3 minutes.
3. Add garlic and Cooking Time: 2 minutes.
4. Add remaining ingredients and lock the lid into place.
5. High-pressure 2 minutes.

6. Use a natural pressure release Directions.
7. Open the lid and transfer into a bowl.
8. Serve with pasta.

396. Delicious Bbq Sauce

Preparation Time: 7 Minutes
Servings: 6
Ingredients:

- ¼ cup coconut oil
- 1 tablespoon molasses
- 1 cup raw cider vinegar
- 2 teaspoons vegan Worcestershire sauce
- 1 teaspoon coconut aminos
- 1 tablespoon Dijon mustard
- 1 good pinch Cayenne pepper
- 1/3 cup coconut sugar

Directions:

1. Heat coconut oil into Instant pot on Sauté.
2. Add remaining ingredients and lock lid into place.
3. Select Manual and high-pressure 5 minutes.
4. Release the pressure with a quick-pressure release Directions.
5. Open the lid and transfer into bowl.
6. Serve or store into fridge.

397. Thai Curry Sauce

Preparation Time: 7 Minutes
Servings: 6
Ingredients:

- 1 teaspoon coconut oil
- 2 ½ cup full-fat coconut milk
- 1 tablespoon mild curry sauce
- 1 cup vegetable stock
- 1 teaspoon coconut aminos
- 2 cloves garlic, minced

- 1 lemongrass stalk, bruised
- 1 tablespoon lime juice
- 4 tablespoons chopped cilantro

Directions:

1. Heat coconut oil in instant pot on Sauté.
2. Add garlic and curry paste and Cooking Time: 30 seconds.
3. Add remaining ingredients, and lock lid into place.
4. Select Manual and High-pressure 4 minutes.
5. Use a natural pressure release Directions.
6. Open the lid and strain into a bowl.
7. Serve or store into a fridge.

398. Sweet Peanut Sauce

Preparation Time: 35 Minutes
Servings: 4
Ingredients:

- 1 cup peanut butter, organic
- ½ cup peanut oil
- 1 teaspoon garlic powder
- 4 tablespoons maple syrup or coconut nectar
- 2 cups water
- 1 teaspoon chili flakes
- 1 tablespoon lime juice
- 1 teaspoon ground cumin
- ½ teaspoon ground fennel
- Salt, to taste

Directions:

1. Combine all ingredients into a food blender.
2. Blend until smooth.
3. Transfer the ingredients into Instant pot.
4. Lock lid into place and select Manual.
5. Low-pressure 30 minutes.

6. Use a natural pressure release Directions.
7. Open the lid and serve sauce.

399. Fast Hollandaise Sauce

Preparation Time: 5 Minutes
Servings: 4
Ingredients:

- ¼ cup fresh lemon juice
- 1 tablespoon nutritional yeast
- 1/3 cup Vegan mayonnaise
- 1 ½ tablespoons Dijon mustard
- 3 tablespoons almond milk
- 1 pinch salt
- 1 pinch black pepper
- 2 cups water

Directions:

1. Pour water into Instant pot and insert trivet.
2. Combine all ingredients into food blender.
3. Blend until smooth. Transfer into heat-proof bowl.
4. Place the bowl onto trivet and lock lid.
5. Select Sauté and adjust heat to More.
6. Steam 3 minutes.
7. Remove from the Instant pot and whisk with a wire whisk until fluffy.
8. Serve.

SNACKS

400. Butter Carrots

Preparation time: 10 minutes
Cooking time: 10 minutes
Total time: 20 minutes
Servings: 04
Ingredients:

- 2 cups baby carrots
- 1 tablespoon brown sugar
- ½ tablespoon vegan butter, melted
- A pinch each salt and black pepper

How to Prepare:
1. Take a baking dish suitable to fit in your air fryer.
2. Toss carrots with sugar, butter, salt and black pepper in the baking dish.
3. Place the dish in the air fryer basket and seal the fryer.
4. Cooking Time: the carrots for 10 minutes at 350 degrees F on air fryer mode.
5. Enjoy.

Nutritional Values:
Calories 119
Total Fat 14 g
Saturated Fat 2 g
Cholesterol 65 mg
Sodium 269 mg
Total Carbs 19 g
Fiber 4 g
Sugar 6 g
Protein 5g

401. Leeks With Butter

Preparation time: 10 minutes
Cooking time: 7 minutes
Total time: 17 minutes
Servings: 04
Ingredients:

- 1 tablespoon vegan butter, melted
- 1 tablespoon lemon juice
- 4 leeks, washed and halved
- Salt and black pepper to taste

How to Prepare:
1. Take a baking dish suitable to fit in your air fryer.
2. Toss the leeks with butter, salt, and black pepper in the dish.
3. Place the dish in the air fryer basket.
4. Seal the fryer and Cooking Time: the carrots for 7 minutes at 350 degrees F on air fryer mode.
5. Add a drizzle of lemon juice.
6. Mix well then serve.

Nutritional Values:
Calories 231
Total Fat 20.1 g
Saturated Fat 2.4 g
Cholesterol 110 mg
Sodium 941 mg
Total Carbs 20.1 g
Fiber 0.9 g
Sugar 1.4 g
Protein 4.6 g

402. Juicy Brussel Sprouts

Preparation time: 10 minutes
Cooking time: 10 minutes
Total time: 20 minutes
Servings: 04
Ingredients:

- 1-pound brussels sprouts, trimmed
- ¼ cup green onions, chopped
- 6 cherry tomatoes, halved
- 1 tablespoon olive oil
- Salt and black pepper to taste

How to Prepare:
1. Take a baking dish suitable to fit in your air fryer.

2. Toss brussels sprouts with salt and black pepper in the dish.
3. Place this dish in the air fryer and seal the fryer.
4. Cooking Time: the sprouts for 10 minutes at 350 degrees F on air fryer mode.
5. Toss these sprouts with green onions, tomatoes, olive oil, salt, and pepper in a salad bowl.
6. Devour.

Nutritional Values:
Calories 361
Total Fat 16.3 g
Saturated Fat 4.9 g
Cholesterol 114 mg
Sodium 515 mg
Total Carbs 29.3 g
Fiber 0.1 g
Sugar 18.2 g
Protein 3.3 g

403. Parsley Potatoes

Preparation time: 10 minutes
Cooking time: 10 minutes
Total time: 20 minutes
Servings: 4
Ingredients:
- 1-pound gold potatoes, sliced
- 2 tablespoons olive oil
- ¼ cup parsley leaves, chopped
- Juice from ½ lemon
- Salt and black pepper to taste

How to Prepare:
1. Take a baking dish suitable to fit in your air fryer.
2. Place the potatoes in it and season them liberally with salt, pepper, olive oil, and lemon juice.
3. Place the baking dish in the air fryer basket and seal it.

4. Cooking Time: the potatoes for 10 minutes at 350 degrees F on air fryer mode.
5. Serve warm with parsley garnishing.
6. Devour.

Nutritional Values:
Calories 205
Total Fat 22.7 g
Saturated Fat 6.1 g
Cholesterol 4 mg
Sodium 227 mg
Total Carbs 26.1 g
Fiber 1.4 g
Sugar 0.9 g
Protein 5.2 g

404. Fried Asparagus

Preparation time: 10 minutes
Cooking time: 8 minutes
Total time: 18 minutes
Servings: 04
Ingredients:
- 2 pounds fresh asparagus, trimmed
- ½ teaspoon oregano, dried
- 4 ounces vegan feta cheese, crumbled
- 4 garlic cloves, minced
- 2 tablespoons parsley, chopped
- ¼ teaspoon red pepper flakes
- ¼ cup olive oil
- Salt and black pepper to the taste
- 1 teaspoon lemon zest
- 1 lemon, juiced

How to Prepare:
1. Combine lemon zest with oregano, pepper flakes, garlic and oil in a large bowl.
2. Add asparagus, salt, pepper, and cheese to the bowl.
3. Toss well to coat then place the asparagus in the air fryer basket.

4. Seal the fryer and Cooking Time: them for 8 minutes at 350 degrees F on Air fryer mode.
5. Garnish with parsley and lemon juice.
6. Enjoy warm.

Nutritional Values:
Calories 201
Total Fat 8.9 g
Saturated Fat 4.5 g
Cholesterol 57 mg
Sodium 340 mg
Total Carbs 24.7 g
Fiber 1.2 g
Sugar 1.3 g
Protein 15.3 g

405. Balsamic Artichokes

Preparation time: 10 minutes
Cooking time: 7 minutes
Total time: 17 minutes
Servings: 04
Ingredients:

- 4 big artichokes, trimmed
- ¼ cup olive oil
- 2 garlic cloves, minced
- 2 tablespoons lemon juice
- 2 teaspoons balsamic vinegar
- 1 teaspoon oregano, dried
- Salt and black pepper to the taste

How to Prepare:
1. Season artichokes liberally with salt and pepper then rub them with half of the lemon juice and oil.
2. Add the artichokes to a baking dish suitable to fit in the air fryer.
3. Place the artichoke dish in the air fryer basket and seal it.
4. Cooking Time: them for 7 minutes at 360 degrees F on air fryer mode.
5. Whisk remaining lemon juice, and oil, vinegar, oregano, garlic, salt and

pepper in a bowl.
6. Pour this mixture over the artichokes and mix them well.
7. Enjoy.

Nutritional Values:
Calories 119
Total Fat 14 g
Saturated Fat 2 g
Cholesterol 65 mg
Sodium 269 mg
Total Carbs 19 g
Fiber 4 g
Sugar 6 g
Protein 5g

406. Tomato Kebabs

Preparation time: 10 minutes
Cooking time: 6 minutes
Total time: 16 minutes
Servings: 04
Ingredients:

- 3 tablespoons balsamic vinegar
- 24 cherry tomatoes
- 2 cups vegan feta cheese, sliced
- 2 tablespoons olive oil
- 3 garlic cloves, minced
- 1 tablespoon thyme, chopped
- Salt and black pepper to the taste

Dressing:

- 2 tablespoons balsamic vinegar
- 4 tablespoons olive oil
- Salt and black pepper to taste

How to Prepare:
1. In a medium bowl combine oil, garlic cloves, thyme, salt, vinegar, and black pepper.
2. Mix well then add the tomatoes and coat them liberally.
3. Thread 6 tomatoes and cheese slices on each skewer alternatively.

4. Place these skewers in the air fryer basket and seal it.
5. Cooking Time: them for 6 minutes on air fryer mode at 360 degrees F.
6. Meanwhile, whisk together the dressing ingredients.
7. Place the cooked skewers on the serving plates.
8. Pour the vinegar dressing over them.
9. Enjoy.

Nutritional Values:
Calories 231
Total Fat 20.1 g
Saturated Fat 2.4 g
Cholesterol 110 mg
Sodium 941 mg
Total Carbs 20.1 g
Fiber 0.9 g
Sugar 1.4 g
Protein 4.6 g

407. Eggplant And Zucchini Snack

Preparation time: 10 minutes
Cooking time: 8 minutes
Total time: 18 minutes
Servings: 04
Ingredients:
- 1 eggplant, cubed
- 3 zucchinis, cubed
- 2 tablespoons lemon juice
- 1 teaspoon oregano, dried
- 3 tablespoons olive oil
- 1 teaspoon thyme, dried
- Salt and black pepper to taste

How to Prepare:
1. Take a baking dish suitable to fit in your air fryer.
2. Combine all ingredients in the baking dish.
3. Place the eggplant dish in the air fryer

basket and seal it.
4. Cooking Time: them for 8 minutes at 360 degrees F on air fryer mode.
5. Enjoy warm.

Nutritional Values:
Calories 361
Total Fat 16.3 g
Saturated Fat 4.9 g
Cholesterol 114 mg
Sodium 515 mg
Total Carbs 29.3 g
Fiber 0.1 g
Sugar 18.2 g
Protein 3.3 g

408. Artichokes With Mayo Sauce

Preparation time: 10 minutes
Cooking time: 6 minutes
Total time: 16 minutes
Servings: 4
Ingredients:
- 2 artichokes, trimmed
- 1 tablespoon lemon juice
- 2 garlic cloves, minced
- A drizzle olive oil
- Sauce:
- 1 cup vegan mayonnaise
- ¼ cup olive oil
- ¼ cup coconut oil
- 3 garlic cloves

How to Prepare:
1. Toss artichokes with lemon juice, oil and 2 garlic cloves in a large bowl.
2. Place the seasoned artichokes in the air fryer basket and seal it.
3. Cooking Time: the artichokes for 6 minutes at 350 degrees on air fryer mode.
4. Blend coconut oil with olive oil, mayonnaise and 3 garlic cloves in a

food processor.

5. Place the artichokes on the serving plates.
6. Pour the mayonnaise mixture over the artichokes.
7. Enjoy fresh.

Nutritional Values:

Calories 205

Total Fat 22.7 g

Saturated Fat 6.1 g

Cholesterol 4 mg

Sodium 227 mg

Total Carbs 26.1 g

Fiber 1.4 g

Sugar 0.9 g

Protein 5.2 g

409. Fried Mustard Greens

Preparation time: 10 minutes

Cooking time: 11 minutes

Total time: 21 minutes

Servings: 04

Ingredients:

- 2 garlic cloves, minced
- 1 tablespoon olive oil
- ½ cup yellow onion, sliced
- 3 tablespoons vegetable stock
- ¼ teaspoon dark sesame oil
- 1-pound mustard greens, torn
- salt and black pepper to the taste

How to Prepare:

1. Take a baking dish suitable to fit in your air fryer.
2. Add oil and place it over the medium heat and sauté onions in it for 5 minutes.
3. Stir in garlic, greens, salt, pepper, and stock.
4. Mix well then place the dish in the air fryer basket.
5. Seal it and Cooking Time: them for 6

minutes at 350 degrees F on air fryer mode.
6. Drizzle sesame oil over the greens.
7. Devour.

Nutritional Values:

Calories 201

Total Fat 8.9 g

Saturated Fat 4.5 g

Cholesterol 57 mg

Sodium 340 mg

Total Carbs 24.7 g

Fiber 1.2 g

Sugar 1.3 g

Protein 15.3 g

410. Cheese Brussels Sprouts

Preparation time: 10 minutes

Cooking time: 8 minutes

Total time: 18 minutes

Servings: 04

Ingredients:

- 1-pound brussels sprouts, washed
- 3 tablespoons vegan parmesan, grated
- Juice from 1 lemon
- 2 tablespoons vegan butter
- Salt and black pepper to the taste

How to Prepare:

1. Spread the brussels sprouts in the air fryer basket.
2. Seal it and Cooking Time: them for 8 minutes at 350 degrees F on air fryer mode.
3. Place a nonstick pan over medium high heat and add butter to melt.
4. Stir in pepper, salt, lemon juice, and brussels sprouts.
5. Mix well then add parmesan.
6. Serve warm.

Nutritional Values:

Calories 119

Total Fat 14 g

Saturated Fat 2 g
Cholesterol 65 mg
Sodium 269 mg
Total Carbs 19 g
Fiber 4 g
Sugar 6 g
Protein 5g

411. Mushroom Stuffed Poblano

Preparation time: 10 minutes
Cooking time: 20 minutes
Total time: 30 minutes
Servings: 10
Ingredients:

- 10 poblano peppers, tops cut off and seeds removed
- 2 teaspoons garlic, minced
- 8 ounces mushrooms, chopped
- ½ cup cilantro, chopped
- 1 white onion, chopped
- 1 tablespoon olive oil
- Salt and black pepper to taste

How to Prepare:
1. Place a nonstick pan over medium heat and add oil.
2. Stir in mushrooms and onion, sauté for 5 minutes.
3. Add salt, black pepper, cilantro and garlic.
4. Stir while cooking for 2 additional minutes then take it off the heat.
5. Divide this mixture in the poblano peppers and stuff them neatly.
6. Place the peppers in the air fryer basket and seal it.
7. Cooking Time: them for 15 minutes at 350 degrees F on air fryer mode.
8. Enjoy.

Nutritional Values:
Calories 231

Total Fat 20.1 g
Saturated Fat 2.4 g
Cholesterol 110 mg
Sodium 941 mg
Total Carbs 20.1 g
Fiber 0.9 g
Sugar 1.4 g
Protein 4.6 g

412. Mushroom Stuffed Tomatoes

Preparation time: 10 minutes
Cooking time: 15 minutes
Total time: 25 minutes
Servings: 04
Ingredients:

- 4 tomatoes, tops removed and pulp removed (reserve for filling
- 1 yellow onion, chopped
- ½ cup mushrooms, chopped
- 1 tablespoon bread crumbs
- 1 tablespoon vegan butter
- ¼ teaspoon caraway seeds
- 1 tablespoon parsley, chopped
- 2 tablespoons celery, chopped
- 1 cup vegan cheese, shredded
- Salt and black pepper to the taste

How to Prepare:
1. Place a pan over medium heat, add butter.
2. When it melts, add onion and celery to sauté for 3 minutes.
3. Stir in mushrooms and tomato pulp.
4. Cooking Time: for 1 minute then add crumbled bread, pepper, salt, cheese, parsley, and caraway seeds.
5. Cooking Time: while stirring for 4 minutes then remove from the heat.
6. After cooling the mixture, stuff it equally in the tomatoes.
7. Place the tomatoes in the air fryer

basket and seal it.

8. Cooking Time: them for 8 minutes at 350 degrees F on air fryer mode.
9. Enjoy.

Nutritional Values:
Calories 361
Total Fat 16.3 g
Saturated Fat 4.9 g
Cholesterol 114 mg
Sodium 515 mg
Total Carbs 29.3 g
Fiber 0.1 g
Sugar 18.2 g
Protein 3.3 g

413. Spinach Stuffed Portobello

Preparation time: 10 minutes
Cooking time: 12 minutes
Total time: 22 minutes
Servings: 4
Ingredients:

- 4 portobello mushrooms, chopped
- 10 basil leaves
- 1 tablespoon parsley
- ¼ cup olive oil
- 8 cherry tomatoes, halved
- 1 cup baby spinach
- 3 garlic cloves, chopped
- 1 cup almonds, chopped
- Salt and black pepper to the taste

How to Prepare:
1. Add all ingredients except mushrooms to a food processor.
2. Blend it all well until smooth then stuff each mushroom cap with the mixture.
3. Place the stuffed mushrooms in the air fryer basket and seal it.
4. Cooking Time: them for 12 minutes at 350 degrees F on air fryer mode.

5. Enjoy.

Nutritional Values:
Calories 205
Total Fat 22.7 g
Saturated Fat 6.1 g
Cholesterol 4 mg
Sodium 227 mg
Total Carbs 26.1 g
Fiber 1.4 g
Sugar 0.9 g
Protein 5.2 g

414. Seasoned Potatoes

Preparation time: 10 minutes
Cooking time: 12 minutes
Total time: 22 minutes
Servings: 04
Ingredients:

- 1 tablespoon coriander seeds
- ½ teaspoon turmeric powder
- ½ teaspoon red chili powder
- 1 teaspoon pomegranate powder
- 1 tablespoon pickled mango, chopped
- 1 tablespoon cumin seeds
- 2 teaspoons fenugreeks, dried
- 5 potatoes, boiled, peeled and cubed
- Salt and black pepper to the taste
- 2 tablespoons olive oil

How to Prepare:
1. Take a baking dish suitable to fit in your air fryer.
2. Add oil, coriander, and cumin seeds to the dish.
3. Place it over medium heat and sauté for 2 minutes.
4. Stir in the rest of the ingredients.
5. Mix well then spread the potatoes in the air fryer basket.
6. Seal it and Cooking Time: them for 10 minutes at 360 degrees F on Air fryer

mode.

7. Serve warm.

Nutritional Values:
Calories 201
Total Fat 8.9 g
Saturated Fat 4.5 g
Cholesterol 57 mg
Sodium 340 mg
Total Carbs 24.7 g
Fiber 1.2 g
Sugar 1.3 g
Protein 15.3 g

415. Black Bean Lime Dip

Preparation Time: 5 minutes
Cooking Time: 6 minutes
Servings: 4
Ingredients:

- 15.5 ounces cooked black beans
- 1 teaspoon minced garlic
- ½ of a lime, juiced
- 1 inch of ginger, grated
- 1/3 teaspoon salt
- 1/3 teaspoon ground black pepper
- 1 tablespoon olive oil

Directions:

1. Take a frying pan, add oil and when hot, add garlic and ginger and Cooking Time: for 1 minute until fragrant.
2. Then add beans, splash with some water and fry for 3 minutes until hot.
3. Season beans with salt and black pepper, drizzle with lime juice, then remove the pan from heat and mash the beans until smooth pasta comes together.
4. Serve the dip with whole-grain breadsticks or vegetables.

Nutrition:
Calories: 374 Cal
Fat: 14 g
Carbs: 46 g
Protein: 15 g
Fiber: 17 g

416. Beetroot Hummus

Preparation Time: 10 minutes
Cooking Time: 60 minutes
Servings: 4
Ingredients:

- 15 ounces cooked chickpeas
- 3 small beets
- 1 teaspoon minced garlic
- 1/2 teaspoon smoked paprika
- 1 teaspoon of sea salt
- 1/4 teaspoon red chili flakes
- 2 tablespoons olive oil
- 1 lemon, juiced
- 2 tablespoon tahini
- 1 tablespoon chopped almonds
- 1 tablespoon chopped cilantro

Directions:

1. Drizzle oil over beets, season with salt, then wrap beets in a foil and bake for 60 minutes at 425 degrees F until tender.
2. When done, let beet cool for 10 minutes, then peel and dice them and place them in a food processor.
3. Add remaining ingredients and pulse for 2 minutes until smooth, tip the hummus in a bowl, drizzle with some more oil, and then serve straight away.

Nutrition:
Calories: 50.1 Cal
Fat: 2.5 g
Carbs: 5 g
Protein: 2 g
Fiber: 1 g

417. Zucchini Hummus

Preparation Time: 5 minutes
Cooking Time: 0 minute
Servings: 8
Ingredients:

- 1 cup diced zucchini
- 1/2 teaspoon sea salt
- 1 teaspoon minced garlic
- 2 teaspoons ground cumin
- 3 tablespoons lemon juice
- 1/3 cup tahini

Directions:

1. Place all the ingredients in a food processor and pulse for 2 minutes until smooth.
2. Tip the hummus in a bowl, drizzle with oil and serve.

Nutrition:
Calories: 65 Cal
Fat: 5 g
Carbs: 3 g
Protein: 2 g
Fiber: 1 g

418. Chipotle And Lime Tortilla Chips

Preparation Time: 10 minutes
Cooking Time: 15 minutes
Servings: 4
Ingredients:

- 12 ounces whole-wheat tortillas
- 4 tablespoons chipotle seasoning
- 1 tablespoon olive oil
- 4 limes, juiced

Directions:

1. Whisk together oil and lime juice, brush it well on tortillas, then sprinkle with chipotle seasoning and bake for 15 minutes at 350 degrees F until crispy, turning halfway.

2. When done, let the tortilla cool for 10 minutes, then break it into chips and serve.

Nutrition:
Calories: 150 Cal
Fat: 7 g
Carbs: 18 g
Protein: 2 g
Fiber: 2 g

419. Carrot And Sweet Potato Fritters

Preparation Time: 10 minutes
Cooking Time: 8 minutes
Servings: 10
Ingredients:

- 1/3 cup quinoa flour
- 1½ cups shredded sweet potato
- 1 cup grated carrot
- 1/3 teaspoon ground black pepper
- 2/3 teaspoon salt
- 2 teaspoons curry powder
- 2 flax eggs
- 2 tablespoons coconut oil

Directions:

1. Place all the ingredients in a bowl, except for oil, stir well until combined and then shape the mixture into ten small patties
2. Take a large pan, place it over medium-high heat, add oil and when it melts, add patties in it and Cooking Time: for 3 minutes per side until browned.
3. Serve straight away

Nutrition:
Calories: 70 Cal
Fat: 3 g
Carbs: 8 g
Protein: 1 g
Fiber: 1 g

420. Tomato And Pesto Toast

Preparation Time: 5 minutes
Cooking Time: 0 minute
Servings: 4
Ingredients:

- 1 small tomato, sliced
- ¼ teaspoon ground black pepper
- 1 tablespoon vegan pesto
- 2 tablespoons hummus
- 1 slice of whole-grain bread, toasted
- Hemp seeds as needed for garnishing

Directions:

1. Spread hummus on one side of the toast, top with tomato slices and then drizzle with pesto.
2. Sprinkle black pepper on the toast along with hemp seeds and then serve straight away.

Nutrition:
Calories: 214 Cal
Fat: 7.2 g
Carbs: 32 g
Protein: 6.5 g
Fiber: 3 g

421. Avocado And Sprout Toast

Preparation Time: 5 minutes
Cooking Time: 0 minute
Servings: 4
Ingredients:

- 1/2 of a medium avocado, sliced
- 1 slice of whole-grain bread, toasted
- 2 tablespoons sprouts
- 2 tablespoons hummus
- ¼ teaspoon lemon zest
- ½ teaspoon hemp seeds
- ¼ teaspoon red pepper flakes

Directions:

1. Spread hummus on one side of the toast and then top with avocado slices and sprouts.
2. Sprinkle with lemon zest, hemp seeds, and red pepper flakes and then serve straight away.

Nutrition:
Calories: 200 Cal
Fat: 10.5 g
Carbs: 22 g
Protein: 7 g
Fiber: 7 g

422. Apple And Honey Toast

Preparation Time: 5 minutes
Cooking Time: 0 minute
Servings: 4
Ingredients:

- ½ of a small apple, cored, sliced
- 1 slice of whole-grain bread, toasted
- 1 tablespoon honey
- 2 tablespoons hummus
- 1/8 teaspoon cinnamon

Directions:

1. Spread hummus on one side of the toast, top with apple slices and then drizzle with honey.
2. Sprinkle cinnamon on it and then serve straight away.

Nutrition:
Calories: 212 Cal
Fat: 7 g
Carbs: 35 g
Protein: 4 g
Fiber: 5.5 g

423. Thai Snack Mix

Preparation Time: 15 minutes
Cooking Time: 90 minutes
Servings: 4
Ingredients:

- 5 cups mixed nuts
- 1 cup chopped dried pineapple

- 1 cup pumpkin seed
- 1 teaspoon garlic powder
- 1 teaspoon onion powder
- 2 teaspoons paprika
- 1 teaspoon of sea salt
- 1/4 cup coconut sugar
- 1/2 teaspoon red chili powder
- 1/2 teaspoon ground black pepper
- 1 tablespoon red pepper flakes
- 1/2 tablespoon red curry powder
- 2 tablespoons soy sauce
- 2 tablespoons coconut oil

Directions:

1. Switch on the slow cooker, add all the ingredients in it except for dried pineapple and red pepper flakes, stir until combined and Cooking Time: for 90 minutes at high heat setting, stirring every 30 minutes.
2. When done, spread the nut mixture on a baking sheet lined with parchment paper and let it cool.
3. Then spread dried pineapple on top, sprinkle with red pepper flakes and serve.

Nutrition:
Calories: 230 Cal
Fat: 17.5 g
Carbs: 11.5 g
Protein: 6.5 g
Fiber: 2 g

424. Zucchini Fritters

Preparation Time: 10 minutes
Cooking Time: 6 minutes
Servings: 12
Ingredients:

- 1/2 cup quinoa flour
- 3 1/2 cups shredded zucchini
- 1/2 cup chopped scallions

- 1/3 teaspoon ground black pepper
- 1 teaspoon salt
- 2 tablespoons coconut oil
- 2 flax eggs

Directions:

1. Squeeze moisture from the zucchini by wrapping it in a cheesecloth and then transfer it to a bowl.
2. Add remaining ingredients, except for oil, stir until combined and then shape the mixture into twelve patties.
3. Take a skillet pan, place it over medium-high heat, add oil and when hot, add patties and Cooking Time: for 3 minutes per side until brown.
4. Serve the patties with favorite vegan sauce.

Nutrition:
Calories: 37 Cal
Fat: 1 g
Carbs: 4 g
Protein: 2 g
Fiber: 1 g

425. Zucchini Chips

Preparation Time: 10 minutes
Cooking Time: 120 minutes
Servings: 4
Ingredients:

- 1 large zucchini, thinly sliced
- 1 teaspoon salt
- 2 tablespoons olive oil

Directions:

1. Pat dry zucchini slices and then spread them in an even layer on a baking sheet lined with parchment sheet.
2. Whisk together salt and oil, brush this mixture over zucchini slices on both sides and then bake for 2 hours or more until brown and crispy.
3. When done, let the chips cool for 10 minutes and then serve straight away.

Nutrition:
Calories: 54 Cal
Fat: 5 g
Carbs: 1 g
Protein: 0 g

426. Rosemary Beet Chips

Preparation Time: 10 minutes
Cooking Time: 20 minutes
Servings: 3
Ingredients:

- 3 large beets, scrubbed, thinly sliced
- 1/8 teaspoon ground black pepper
- ¼ teaspoon of sea salt
- 3 sprigs of rosemary, leaves chopped
- 4 tablespoons olive oil

Directions:

1. Spread beet slices in a single layer between two large baking sheets, brush the slices with oil, then season with spices and rosemary, toss until well coated, and bake for 20 minutes at 375 degrees F until crispy, turning halfway.
2. When done, let the chips cool for 10 minutes and then serve.

Nutrition:
Calories: 79 Cal
Fat: 4.7 g
Carbs: 8.6 g
Protein: 1.5 g
Fiber: 2.5 g

427. Quinoa Broccoli Tots

Preparation Time: 10 minutes
Cooking Time: 20 minutes
Servings: 16
Ingredients:

- 2 tablespoons quinoa flour
- 2 cups steamed and chopped broccoli florets
- 1/2 cup nutritional yeast
- 1 teaspoon garlic powder
- 1 teaspoon miso paste
- 2 flax eggs
- 2 tablespoons hummus

Directions:

1. Place all the ingredients in a bowl, stir until well combined, and then shape the mixture into sixteen small balls.
2. Arrange the balls on a baking sheet lined with parchment paper, spray with oil and bake at 400 degrees F for 20 minutes until brown, turning halfway.
3. When done, let the tots cool for 10 minutes and then serve straight away.

Nutrition:
Calories: 19 Cal
Fat: 0 g
Carbs: 2 g
Protein: 1 g
Fiber: 0.5 g

428. Spicy Roasted Chickpeas

Preparation Time: 10 minutes
Cooking Time: 20 minutes
Servings: 6
Ingredients:

- 30 ounces cooked chickpeas
- ½ teaspoon salt
- 2 teaspoons mustard powder
- ½ teaspoon cayenne pepper
- 2 tablespoons olive oil

Directions:

1. Place all the ingredients in a bowl and stir until well coated and then spread the chickpeas in an even layer on a baking sheet greased with oil.
2. Bake the chickpeas for 20 minutes at 400 degrees F until golden brown and crispy and then serve straight away.

Nutrition:
Calories: 187.1 Cal
Fat: 7.4 g
Carbs: 24.2 g
Protein: 7.3 g
Fiber: 6.3 g

429. Nacho Kale Chips

Preparation Time: 10 minutes
Cooking Time: 14 hours
Servings: 10
Ingredients:

- 2 bunches of curly kale
- 2 cups cashews, soaked, drained
- 1/2 cup chopped red bell pepper
- 1 teaspoon garlic powder
- 1 teaspoon salt
- 2 tablespoons red chili powder
- 1/2 teaspoon smoked paprika
- 1/2 cup nutritional yeast
- 1 teaspoon cayenne
- 3 tablespoons lemon juice
- 3/4 cup water

Directions:

1. Place all the ingredients except for kale in a food processor and pulse for 2 minutes until smooth.
2. Place kale in a large bowl, pour in the blended mixture, mix until coated, and dehydrate for 14 hours at 120 degrees F until crispy.
3. If dehydrator is not available, spread kale between two baking sheets and bake for 90 minutes at 225 degrees F until crispy, flipping halfway.
4. When done, let chips cool for 15 minutes and then serve.

Nutrition:
Calories: 191 Cal
Fat: 12 g
Carbs: 16 g
Protein: 9 g
Fiber: 2 g

430. Red Salsa

Preparation Time: 10 minutes
Cooking Time: 0 minute
Servings: 8
Ingredients:

- 30 ounces diced fire-roasted tomatoes
- 4 tablespoons diced green chilies
- 1 medium jalapeño pepper, deseeded
- 1/2 cup chopped green onion
- 1 cup chopped cilantro
- 1 teaspoon minced garlic
- ½ teaspoon of sea salt
- 1 teaspoon ground cumin
- ¼ teaspoon stevia
- 3 tablespoons lime juice

Directions:

1. Place all the ingredients in a food processor and process for 2 minutes until smooth.
2. Tip the salsa in a bowl, taste to adjust seasoning and then serve.

Nutrition:
Calories: 71 Cal
Fat: 0.2 g
Carbs: 19 g
Protein: 2 g
Fiber: 4.1 g

431. Tomato Hummus

Preparation Time: 5 minutes
Cooking Time: 0 minute
Servings: 4
Ingredients:

- 1/4 cup sun-dried tomatoes, without oil
- 1 ½ cups cooked chickpeas
- 1 teaspoon minced garlic
- 1/2 teaspoon salt
- 2 tablespoons sesame oil
- 1 tablespoon lemon juice
- 1 tablespoon olive oil
- 1/4 cup of water

Directions:

1. Place all the ingredients in a food processor and process for 2 minutes until smooth.
2. Tip the hummus in a bowl, drizzle with more oil, and then serve straight away.

Nutrition:
Calories: 122.7 Cal
Fat: 4.1 g
Carbs: 17.8 g
Protein: 5.1 g
Fiber: 3.5 g

432. Marinated Mushrooms

Preparation Time: 10 minutes
Cooking Time: 7 minutes
Servings: 6
Ingredients:

- 12 ounces small button mushrooms
- 1 teaspoon minced garlic
- 1/4 teaspoon dried thyme
- 1/2 teaspoon sea salt
- 1/2 teaspoon dried basil
- 1/2 teaspoon red pepper flakes
- 1/4 teaspoon dried oregano
- 1/2 teaspoon maple syrup
- 1/4 cup apple cider vinegar
- 1/4 cup and 1 teaspoon olive oil
- 2 tablespoons chopped parsley

Directions:

1. Take a skillet pan, place it over medium-high heat, add 1 teaspoon oil and when hot, add mushrooms and Cooking Time: for 5 minutes until golden brown.
2. Meanwhile, prepare the marinade and for this, place remaining ingredients in a bowl and whisk until combined.
3. When mushrooms have cooked, transfer them into the bowl of marinade and toss until well coated.
4. Serve straight away

Nutrition:
Calories: 103 Cal
Fat: 9 g
Carbs: 2 g
Protein: 1 g

433. Hummus Quesadillas

Preparation Time: 5 minutes
Cooking Time: 15 minutes
Servings: 1
Ingredients:

- 1 tortilla, whole wheat
- 1/4 cup diced roasted red peppers
- 1 cup baby spinach
- 1/3 teaspoon minced garlic
- ¼ teaspoon salt
- ¼ teaspoon ground black pepper
- 1/4 teaspoon olive oil
- 1/4 cup hummus
- Oil as needed

Directions:

1. Place a large pan over medium heat, add oil and when hot, add red peppers and garlic, season with salt and black

pepper and Cooking Time: for 3 minutes until sauté.

2. Then stir in spinach, Cooking Time: for 1 minute, remove the pan from heat and transfer the mixture in a bowl.

3. Prepare quesadilla and for this, spread hummus on one-half of the tortilla, then spread spinach mixture on it, cover the filling with the other half of the tortilla and Cooking Time: in a pan for 3 minutes per side until browned.

4. When done, cut the quesadilla into wedges and serve.

Nutrition:

Calories: 187 Cal

Fat: 9 g

Carbs: 16.3 g

Protein: 10.4 g

Fiber: 0 g

434. Nacho Cheese Sauce

Preparation Time: 5 minutes

Cooking Time: 10 minutes

Servings: 4

Ingredients:

- 3 tablespoons flour
- 1/4 teaspoon garlic salt
- 1/4 teaspoon salt
- 1/2 teaspoon cumin
- 1/4 teaspoon paprika
- 1 teaspoon red chili powder
- 1/8 teaspoon cayenne powder
- 1 cup vegan cashew yogurt
- 1 1/4 cups vegetable broth

Directions:

1. Take a small saucepan, place it over medium heat, pour in vegetable broth, and bring it to a boil.

2. Then whisk together flour and yogurt,

add to the boiling broth, stir in all the spices, switch heat to medium-low level and Cooking Time: for 5 minutes until thickened.

3. Serve straight away.

Nutrition:

Calories: 282 Cal

Fat: 1 g

Carbs: 63 g

Protein: 3 g

Fiber: 12 g

435. Avocado Tomato Bruschetta

Preparation Time: 10 minutes

Cooking Time: 0 minute

Servings: 4

Ingredients:

- 3 slices of whole-grain bread
- 6 chopped cherry tomatoes
- ½ of sliced avocado
- ½ teaspoon minced garlic
- ½ teaspoon ground black pepper
- 2 tablespoons chopped basil
- ½ teaspoon of sea salt
- 1 teaspoon balsamic vinegar

Directions:

1. Place tomatoes in a bowl, and then stir in vinegar until mixed. Top bread slices with avocado slices, then top evenly with tomato mixture, garlic and basil, and season with salt and black pepper.

2. Serve straight away

Nutrition:

Calories: 131 Cal

Fat: 7.3 g

Carbs: 15 g

Protein: 2.8 g

Fiber: 3.2 g

436. Butter Carrots

Preparation time: 10 minutes
Cooking time: 10 minutes
Total time: 20 minutes
Servings: 04
Ingredients:

- 2 cups baby carrots
- 1 tablespoon brown sugar
- ½ tablespoon vegan butter, melted
- A pinch each salt and black pepper

How to Prepare:
1. Take a baking dish suitable to fit in your air fryer.
2. Toss carrots with sugar, butter, salt and black pepper in the baking dish.
3. Place the dish in the air fryer basket and seal the fryer.
4. Cooking Time: the carrots for 10 minutes at 350 degrees F on air fryer mode.
5. Enjoy.

Nutritional Values:
Calories 119
Total Fat 14 g
Saturated Fat 2 g
Cholesterol 65 mg
Sodium 269 mg
Total Carbs 19 g
Fiber 4 g
Sugar 6 g
Protein 5g

437. Leeks With Butter

Preparation time: 10 minutes
Cooking time: 7 minutes
Total time: 17 minutes
Servings: 04
Ingredients:

- 1 tablespoon vegan butter, melted
- 1 tablespoon lemon juice
- 4 leeks, washed and halved
- Salt and black pepper to taste

How to Prepare:
1. Take a baking dish suitable to fit in your air fryer.
2. Toss the leeks with butter, salt, and black pepper in the dish.
3. Place the dish in the air fryer basket.
4. Seal the fryer and Cooking Time: the carrots for 7 minutes at 350 degrees F on air fryer mode.
5. Add a drizzle of lemon juice.
6. Mix well then serve.

Nutritional Values:
Calories 231
Total Fat 20.1 g
Saturated Fat 2.4 g
Cholesterol 110 mg
Sodium 941 mg
Total Carbs 20.1 g
Fiber 0.9 g
Sugar 1.4 g
Protein 4.6 g

438. Juicy Brussel Sprouts

Preparation time: 10 minutes
Cooking time: 10 minutes
Total time: 20 minutes
Servings: 04
Ingredients:

- 1-pound brussels sprouts, trimmed
- ¼ cup green onions, chopped
- 6 cherry tomatoes, halved
- 1 tablespoon olive oil
- Salt and black pepper to taste

How to Prepare:
1. Take a baking dish suitable to fit in your air fryer.
2. Toss brussels sprouts with salt and black pepper in the dish.
3. Place this dish in the air fryer and seal

the fryer.

4. Cooking Time: the sprouts for 10 minutes at 350 degrees F on air fryer mode.
5. Toss these sprouts with green onions, tomatoes, olive oil, salt, and pepper in a salad bowl.
6. Devour.

Nutritional Values:
Calories 361
Total Fat 16.3 g
Saturated Fat 4.9 g
Cholesterol 114 mg
Sodium 515 mg
Total Carbs 29.3 g
Fiber 0.1 g
Sugar 18.2 g
Protein 3.3 g

439. Parsley Potatoes

Preparation time: 10 minutes
Cooking time: 10 minutes
Total time: 20 minutes
Servings: 4
Ingredients:

- 1-pound gold potatoes, sliced
- 2 tablespoons olive oil
- ¼ cup parsley leaves, chopped
- Juice from ½ lemon
- Salt and black pepper to taste

How to Prepare:
1. Take a baking dish suitable to fit in your air fryer.
2. Place the potatoes in it and season them liberally with salt, pepper, olive oil, and lemon juice.
3. Place the baking dish in the air fryer basket and seal it.
4. Cooking Time: the potatoes for 10 minutes at 350 degrees F on air fryer mode.

5. Serve warm with parsley garnishing.
6. Devour.

Nutritional Values:
Calories 205
Total Fat 22.7 g
Saturated Fat 6.1 g
Cholesterol 4 mg
Sodium 227 mg
Total Carbs 26.1 g
Fiber 1.4 g
Sugar 0.9 g
Protein 5.2 g

440. Fried Asparagus

Preparation time: 10 minutes
Cooking time: 8 minutes
Total time: 18 minutes
Servings: 04
Ingredients:

- 2 pounds fresh asparagus, trimmed
- ½ teaspoon oregano, dried
- 4 ounces vegan feta cheese, crumbled
- 4 garlic cloves, minced
- 2 tablespoons parsley, chopped
- ¼ teaspoon red pepper flakes
- ¼ cup olive oil
- Salt and black pepper to the taste
- 1 teaspoon lemon zest
- 1 lemon, juiced

How to Prepare:
1. Combine lemon zest with oregano, pepper flakes, garlic and oil in a large bowl.
2. Add asparagus, salt, pepper, and cheese to the bowl.
3. Toss well to coat then place the asparagus in the air fryer basket.
4. Seal the fryer and Cooking Time: them for 8 minutes at 350 degrees F on Air fryer mode.
5. Garnish with parsley and lemon juice.

6. Enjoy warm.

Nutritional Values:
Calories 201
Total Fat 8.9 g
Saturated Fat 4.5 g
Cholesterol 57 mg
Sodium 340 mg
Total Carbs 24.7 g
Fiber 1.2 g
Sugar 1.3 g
Protein 15.3 g

441. Balsamic Artichokes

Preparation time: 10 minutes
Cooking time: 7 minutes
Total time: 17 minutes
Servings: 04
Ingredients:
- 4 big artichokes, trimmed
- ¼ cup olive oil
- 2 garlic cloves, minced
- 2 tablespoons lemon juice
- 2 teaspoons balsamic vinegar
- 1 teaspoon oregano, dried
- Salt and black pepper to the taste

How to Prepare:
1. Season artichokes liberally with salt and pepper then rub them with half of the lemon juice and oil.
2. Add the artichokes to a baking dish suitable to fit in the air fryer.
3. Place the artichoke dish in the air fryer basket and seal it.
4. Cooking Time: them for 7 minutes at 360 degrees F on air fryer mode.
5. Whisk remaining lemon juice, and oil, vinegar, oregano, garlic, salt and pepper in a bowl.
6. Pour this mixture over the artichokes and mix them well.
7. Enjoy.

Nutritional Values:
Calories 119
Total Fat 14 g
Saturated Fat 2 g
Cholesterol 65 mg
Sodium 269 mg
Total Carbs 19 g
Fiber 4 g
Sugar 6 g
Protein 5g

442. Tomato Kebabs

Preparation time: 10 minutes
Cooking time: 6 minutes
Total time: 16 minutes
Servings: 04
Ingredients:
- 3 tablespoons balsamic vinegar
- 24 cherry tomatoes
- 2 cups vegan feta cheese, sliced
- 2 tablespoons olive oil
- 3 garlic cloves, minced
- 1 tablespoon thyme, chopped
- Salt and black pepper to the taste

Dressing:
- 2 tablespoons balsamic vinegar
- 4 tablespoons olive oil
- Salt and black pepper to taste

How to Prepare:
1. In a medium bowl combine oil, garlic cloves, thyme, salt, vinegar, and black pepper.
2. Mix well then add the tomatoes and coat them liberally.
3. Thread 6 tomatoes and cheese slices on each skewer alternatively.
4. Place these skewers in the air fryer basket and seal it.
5. Cooking Time: them for 6 minutes on air fryer mode at 360 degrees F.
6. Meanwhile, whisk together the

dressing ingredients.

7. Place the cooked skewers on the serving plates.
8. Pour the vinegar dressing over them.
9. Enjoy.

Nutritional Values:
Calories 231
Total Fat 20.1 g
Saturated Fat 2.4 g
Cholesterol 110 mg
Sodium 941 mg
Total Carbs 20.1 g
Fiber 0.9 g
Sugar 1.4 g
Protein 4.6 g

Calories 361
Total Fat 16.3 g
Saturated Fat 4.9 g
Cholesterol 114 mg
Sodium 515 mg
Total Carbs 29.3 g
Fiber 0.1 g
Sugar 18.2 g
Protein 3.3 g

443. Eggplant And Zucchini Snack

Preparation time: 10 minutes
Cooking time: 8 minutes
Total time: 18 minutes
Servings: 04
Ingredients:

- 1 eggplant, cubed
- 3 zucchinis, cubed
- 2 tablespoons lemon juice
- 1 teaspoon oregano, dried
- 3 tablespoons olive oil
- 1 teaspoon thyme, dried
- Salt and black pepper to taste

How to Prepare:

1. Take a baking dish suitable to fit in your air fryer.
2. Combine all ingredients in the baking dish.
3. Place the eggplant dish in the air fryer basket and seal it.
4. Cooking Time: them for 8 minutes at 360 degrees F on air fryer mode.
5. Enjoy warm.

Nutritional Values:

DESSERT RECIPES

444. Chocolate Brownies

Preparation time: 5 minutes
Cooking Time: time: 20 minutes
Servings: 4
Ingredients:

- 2 tablespoons cocoa powder
- 1 scoop protein powder
- 1 cup bananas, over-ripe
- ½ cup almond butter, melted

Directions:
Preheat the oven to 350° Fahrenheit. Spray the brownie pan with cooking spray. Add all ingredients in your blender and blend until smooth. Pour the batter into the prepared pan and bake in preheated oven for 20 minutes. Serve and enjoy!
Nutrition:
Calories: 82
Sugars: 5 g
Fat: 2.1 g
Carbohydrates: 11.4 g
Cholesterol: 16 mg
Protein: 6.9 g

445. Almond Butter Fudge

Preparation time: 15 minutes
Cooking Time: time: 2 minutes
Servings: 8
Ingredients:

- 2 ½ tablespoons coconut oil
- 2 ½ tablespoons honey
- ½ cup almond butter

Directions:
Combine coconut oil and almond butter in a saucepan and warm for 2 minutes or until melted. Add honey and stir. Pour the mixture into candy container and store in the fridge until set. Serve and enjoy!

Nutrition:
Calories: 63
Carbohydrates: 5.6 g
Fat: 4.8 g
Sugars: 5.4 g
Cholesterol: 0 mg
Protein: 0.2 g

446. White Chocolate Fat Bomb

Preparation time: 5 minutes
Cooking Time: time: 2 minutes
Servings: 8
Ingredients:

- 4 tablespoons butter
- 4 tablespoons coconut oil
- 4 tablespoons erythritol, powdered
- 4-ounces cocoa butter
- ¼ teaspoon salt
- ¼ teaspoon Stevia
- ½ teaspoon vanilla extract
- ½ cup walnuts, chopped

Directions:
Add your cocoa butter and coconut oil into a pan over medium heat for 2 minutes or until melted, then remove from heat. Add Stevia, vanilla extract, erythritol, salt, and walnuts. Mix well to combine. Pour mixture into silicone mold and place in the fridge for an hour. Serve and enjoy!
Nutrition:
Calories: 265
Fat: 20.2 g
Carbohydrates: 0.8 g
Protein: 0.9 g
Fiber: 0.5
Cholesterol: 15 mg

447. Brownie Balls

Preparation time: 20 minutes
Servings: 12
Ingredients:

- 6 dates, pitted
- ¼ cup chocolate chips
- ½ cup almond meal
- 2 tablespoons coconut butter
- 2 teaspoons vanilla extract

Directions:
Add your dates to your food processor and pulse for 3 minutes. Add all remaining ingredients except chocolate chips. Pulse until well combined. Add chocolate chips and pulse for 2 times. Form dough into 12 balls and place into the fridge for 1 hour. Serve and enjoy!
Nutrition:
Calories: 86
Fat: 6 g
Cholesterol: 1 mg
Carbohydrates: 7.3 g
Protein: 1.5 g

448. Peanut Butter Fudge

Preparation time: 15 minutes
Cooking Time: time: 2 minutes
Servings: 20
Ingredients:

- 12-ounces peanut butter, smooth
- 4 tablespoons maple syrup
- 4 tablespoons coconut cream
- 3 tablespoons coconut oil
- Pinch of salt

Directions:
Line baking tray with parchment paper. Melt the coconut and maple syrup in a pan over low heat for about 2 minutes or until melted. Add peanut butter, coconut cream, and salt into the pan, stir well. Pour fudge mixture into the prepared baking dish and place in the fridge for an hour. Cut into pieces serve and enjoy!
Nutrition:
Calories: 135
Carbohydrates: 6.2 g
Sugar: 4.1 g
Cholesterol: 0 mg
Fat: 11.3 g
Protein: 4.3 g

DESSERTS AND DRINKS

449. Oatmeal Raisin Muffins

Preparation time: 10 minutes
Cooking time: 35 minutes
Total time: 45 minutes
Servings: 12
Ingredients:

- 2½ cups rolled oats
- ½ cup oat flour
- 1 teaspoon baking powder
- ½ teaspoon baking soda
- ½ teaspoon salt
- 1 tablespoon cinnamon
- ½ teaspoon ground nutmeg
- 4 ripe bananas, mashed
- 1 apple, grated
- ½ cup almond milk
- 2 teaspoons vanilla extract
- ½ cup raisins
- ½ cup chopped walnuts

How to Prepare:

1. Preheat your oven to 350 degrees F.
2. Whisk the dry ingredients in a mixing bowl, and wet ingredients in a separate bowl.
3. Beat the two mixtures together until smooth.
4. Fold in apples, walnuts and raisins, give it a gentle stir.
5. Line a muffin tray with muffin cups and evenly divide the muffin batter among the cups.
6. Bake for nearly 35 minutes and serve.

Nutritional Values:
Calories 398
Total Fat 6 g
Saturated Fat 7 g
Cholesterol 632 mg
Sodium 497 mg
Total Carbs 91 g
Fiber 3 g
Sugar 83 g
Protein 2 g

450. Applesauce Muffins

Preparation time: 10 minutes
Cooking time: 25 minutes
Total time: 35 minutes
Servings: 12
Ingredients:

- 2 cups whole wheat flour
- 1 teaspoon baking powder
- 1 teaspoon baking soda
- ½ teaspoon salt
- 1 teaspoon cinnamon
- ½ teaspoon ground allspice
- ½ cup brown sugar
- 15 ounces apple sauce
- ½ cup almond milk
- 1 teaspoon vanilla
- 1 teaspoon apple cider vinegar
- ½ cup raisins
- ½ cup apple, diced

How to Prepare:

1. Preheat your oven to 350 degrees F.
2. Separately, whisk together the dry ingredients in one bowl and wet ingredients in another bowl.
3. Beat the two mixture together until smooth.
4. Fold in apples and raisins, give it a gentle stir.
5. Line a muffin tray with muffin cups and evenly divide the muffin batter among the cups.
6. Bake for nearly 25 minutes and serve.

Nutritional Values:
Calories 232
Total Fat 8.9 g
Saturated Fat 4.5 g
Cholesterol 57 mg
Sodium 340 mg
Total Carbs 24.7 g
Fiber 1.2 g
Sugar 12.3 g
Protein 5.3 g

451. Banana Cinnamon Muffins

Preparation time: 10 minutes
Cooking time: 22 minutes
Total time: 32 minutes
Servings: 12
Ingredients:

- 3 very ripe bananas, mashed
- ½ cup vanilla almond milk
- 1 cup sugar
- 2 cups flour
- 1 teaspoon baking soda
- ½ teaspoon cinnamon
- ¼ teaspoon salt

How to Prepare:
1. Preheat your oven to 350 degrees F.
2. Separately, whisk together the dry ingredients in one bowl and the wet ingredients in another bowl.
3. Beat the two mixtures together until smooth.
4. Line a muffin tray with muffin cups and evenly divide the muffin batter among the cups.
5. Bake for 22 minutes and serve.

Nutritional Values:
Calories 427
Total Fat 31.1 g
Saturated Fat 4.2 g
Cholesterol 123 mg
Sodium 86 mg

Total Carbs 29 g
Sugar 12.4 g
Fiber 19.8 g
Protein 3.5 g

452. Cashew Oat Muffins

Preparation time: 10 minutes
Cooking time: 22 minutes
Total time: 32 minutes
Servings: 12
Ingredients:

- 3 cups rolled oats
- ¾ cup raw cashews
- ¼ cup maple syrup
- ¼ cup sugar
- 1 teaspoon vanilla extract
- ½ teaspoon salt
- 1½ teaspoon baking soda
- 2 cups water

How to Prepare:
1. Preheat your oven to 375 degrees F.
2. Separately, whisk together the dry ingredients in one bowl and the wet ingredients in another bowl.
3. Beat the two mixtures together until smooth.
4. Fold in cashews and give it a gentle stir.
5. Line a muffin tray with muffin cups and evenly divide the muffin batter among the cups.
6. Bake for 22 minutes and serve.

Nutritional Values:
Calories 398
Total Fat 13.8 g
Saturated Fat 5.1 g
Cholesterol 200 mg
Sodium 272 mg
Total Carbs 53.6 g
Fiber 1 g
Sugar 12.3 g

Protein 1.8 g

453. Banana Walnut Muffins

Preparation time: 10 minutes
Cooking time: 18 minutes
Total time: 28 minutes
Servings: 12
Ingredients:

- 4 large pitted dates, boiled
- 1 cup almond milk
- 2 tablespoons lemon juice
- 2½ cups rolled oats
- 1 teaspoon baking powder
- 1 teaspoon baking soda
- 1 teaspoon cinnamon
- ¼ teaspoon nutmeg
- ⅛ teaspoon salt
- 1½ cups mashed banana
- ¼ cup maple syrup
- 1 tablespoon vanilla extract
- 1 cup walnuts, chopped

How to Prepare:

1. Preheat your oven to 350 degrees F.
2. Separately, whisk together the dry ingredients in one bowl and the wet ingredients in another bowl.
3. Beat the two mixtures together until smooth.
4. Fold in walnuts and give it a gentle stir.
5. Line a muffin tray with muffin cups and evenly divide the muffin batter among the cups.
6. Bake for 18 minutes and serve.

Nutritional Values:
Calories 265
Total Fat 14 g
Saturated Fat 7 g
Cholesterol 632 mg
Sodium 497 mg

Total Carbs 36 g
Fiber 3 g
Sugar 10 g
Protein 5 g

454. Carrot Flaxseed Muffins

Preparation time: 10 minutes
Cooking time: 20 minutes
Total time: 30 minutes
Servings: 12
Ingredients:

- 2 tablespoons ground flax
- 5 tablespoons water
- ¾ cup almond milk
- ¾ cup applesauce
- ½ cup maple syrup
- 1 teaspoon vanilla extract
- 1½ cups whole wheat flour
- ½ cup rolled oats
- 1 teaspoon baking soda
- 1½ teaspoons baking powder
- ½ teaspoon salt
- 1 teaspoon ground cinnamon
- ¼ teaspoon ground ginger
- 1 cup grated carrot

How to Prepare:

1. Whisk flaxseed with water in a bowl and leave it for 10 minutes
2. Preheat your oven to 350 degrees F.
3. Separately, whisk together the dry ingredients in one bowl and the wet ingredients in another bowl.
4. Beat the two mixtures together until smooth.
5. Fold in flaxseed and carrots, give it a gentle stir.
6. Line a muffin tray with muffin cups and evenly divide the muffin batter among the cups.
7. Bake for 20 minutes and serve.

Nutritional Values:
Calories 172
Total Fat 11.8 g
Saturated Fat 4.4 g
Cholesterol 62 mg
Sodium 871 mg
Total Carbs 45.8 g
Fiber 0.6 g
Sugar 2.3 g
Protein 4 g

455. Chocolate Peanut Fat Bombs

Preparation time: 10 minutes
Cooking time: 1 hour 1 minute
Total time: 1 hour and 11 minutes
Servings: 12
Ingredients:

- ½ cup coconut butter
- 1 cup plus 2 tablespoons peanut butter
- 5 tablespoons cocoa powder
- 2 teaspoons maple syrup

How to Prepare:
1. In a bowl, combine all the ingredients.
2. Melt them in the microwave for 1 minute.
3. Mix well then divide the mixture into silicone molds.
4. Freeze them for 1 hour to set.
5. Serve.

Nutritional Values:
Calories 246
Total Fat 7.4 g
Saturated Fat 4.6 g
Cholesterol 105 mg
Sodium 353 mg
Total Carbs 29.4 g
Sugar 6.5 g
Fiber 2.7 g
Protein 7.2 g

456. Protein Fat Bombs

Preparation time: 10 minutes
Cooking time: 1 hour
Total time: 1 hour and 10 minutes
Servings: 12
Ingredients:

- 1 cup coconut oil
- 1 cup peanut butter, melted
- ½ cup cocoa powder
- ¼ cup plant-based protein powder
- 1 pinch of salt
- 2 cups unsweetened shredded coconut

How to Prepare:
1. In a bowl, add all the ingredients except coconut shreds.
2. Mix well then make small balls out of this mixture and place them into silicone molds.
3. Freeze for 1 hour to set.
4. Roll the balls in the coconut shreds
5. Serve.

Nutritional Values:
Calories 293
Total Fat 16 g
Saturated Fat 2.3 g
Cholesterol 75 mg
Sodium 386 mg
Total Carbs 25.2 g
Sugar 2.6 g
Fiber 1.9 g
Protein 4.2 g

457. Mojito Fat Bombs

Preparation time: 10 minutes
Cooking time: 1 hour and 1 minute
Total time: 1 hour and 11 minutes
Servings: 12
Ingredients:

- ¾ cup hulled hemp seeds
- ½ cup coconut oil

- 1 cup fresh mint
- ½ teaspoon mint extract
- Juice & zest of two limes
- ¼ teaspoon stevia

How to Prepare:
1. In a bowl, combine all the ingredients.
2. Melt in the microwave for 1 minute.
3. Mix well then divide the mixture into silicone molds.
4. Freeze them for 1 hour to set.
5. Serve.

Nutritional Values:
Calories 319
Total Fat 10.6 g
Saturated Fat 3.1 g
Cholesterol 131 mg
Sodium 834 mg
Total Carbs 31.4 g
Fiber 0.2 g
Sugar 0.3 g
Protein 4.6 g

458. Apple Pie Bites

Preparation time: 10 minutes
Cooking time: 1 hour
Total time: 1 hour and 10 minutes
Servings: 12
Ingredients:
- 1 cup walnuts, chopped
- ½ cup coconut oil
- ¼ cup ground flax seeds
- ½ ounce freeze dried apples
- 1 teaspoon vanilla extract
- 1 teaspoon cinnamon
- Liquid stevia, to taste

How to Prepare:
1. In a bowl add all the ingredients.
2. Mix well then roll the mixture into small balls.
3. Freeze them for 1 hour to set.

4. Serve.
Nutritional Values:
Calories 211
Total Fat 25.5 g
Saturated Fat 12.4 g
Cholesterol 69 mg
Sodium 58 mg
Total Carbs 32.4 g
Fiber 0.7 g
Sugar 0.3 g
Protein 1.4 g

459. Coconut Fat Bombs

Preparation time: 10 minutes
Cooking time: 1 hour and 1 minute
Total time: 1 hour and 11 minutes
Servings: 12
Ingredients:
- 1 can coconut milk
- ¾ cup coconut oil
- 1 cup coconut flakes
- 20 drops liquid stevia

How to Prepare:
1. In a bowl combine all the ingredients.
2. Melt in a microwave for 1 minute.
3. Mix well then divide the mixture into silicone molds.
4. Freeze them for 1 hour to set.
5. Serve.
Nutritional Values:
Calories 119
Total Fat 14 g
Saturated Fat 2 g
Cholesterol 65 mg
Sodium 269 mg
Total Carbs 19 g
Fiber 4 g
Sugar 6 g
Protein 5g

460. Peach Popsicles

Preparation time: 10 minutes
Cooking time: 2 hours
Total time: 2 hours and 10 minutes
Servings: 2
Ingredients:

- 2½ cups peaches, peeled and pitted
- 2 tablespoons agave
- ¾ cup coconut cream

How to Prepare:
1. In a blender, blend all the ingredients for popsicles until smooth.
2. Divide the popsicle blend into the popsicle molds.
3. Insert the popsicles sticks and close the molds.
4. Place the molds in the freezer for 2 hours to set.
5. Serve.

Nutritional Values:
Calories 231
Total Fat 20.1 g
Saturated Fat 2.4 g
Cholesterol 110 mg
Sodium 941 mg
Total Carbs 20.1 g
Fiber 0.9 g
Sugar 1.4 g
Protein 4.6 g

461. Green Popsicle

Preparation time: 10 minutes
Cooking time: 2 hours
Total time: 2 hours and 10 minutes
Servings: 4
Ingredients:

- 1 ripe avocado, peeled and pitted
- 1 cup fresh spinach
- 1 can (13.5 ouncefull fat coconut milk
- ¼ cup lime juice

- 2 tablespoons maple syrup
- 1 teaspoon vanilla extract

How to Prepare:
1. In a blender, blend all the ingredients for popsicles until smooth.
2. Divide the popsicle blend into the popsicle molds.
3. Insert the popsicles sticks and close the molds.
4. Place the molds in the freezer for 2 hours to set.
5. Serve.

Nutritional Values:
Calories 361
Total Fat 16.3 g
Saturated Fat 4.9 g
Cholesterol 114 mg
Sodium 515 mg
Total Carbs 29.3 g
Fiber 0.1 g
Sugar 18.2 g
Protein 3.3 g

462. Strawberry Coconut Popsicles

Preparation time: 10 minutes
Cooking time: 2 hours
Total time: 2 hours and 10 minutes
Servings: 2
Ingredients:

- 2 medium bananas, sliced
- 1 can coconut milk
- 1 cup strawberries
- 3 tablespoons maple syrup

How to Prepare:
1. In a blender, blend all the ingredients for popsicles until smooth.
2. Divide the popsicle blend into the popsicle molds.
3. Insert the popsicles sticks and close the molds.

4. Place the molds in the freezer for 2 hours to set.
5. Serve.

Nutritional Values:
Calories 205
Total Fat 22.7 g
Saturated Fat 6.1 g
Cholesterol 4 mg
Sodium 227 mg
Total Carbs 26.1 g
Fiber 1.4 g
Sugar 0.9 g
Protein 5.2 g

463. Fudge Popsicles

Preparation time: 10 minutes
Cooking time: 2 hours
Total time: 2 hours and 10 minutes
Servings: 2
Ingredients:

- 1 cup almond milk
- 3 ripe bananas
- 3 tablespoon cocoa powder
- 1 tablespoon almond butter

How to Prepare:
1. In a blender, blend all the ingredients for popsicles until smooth.
2. Divide the popsicle blend into the popsicle molds.
3. Insert the popsicles sticks and close the molds.
4. Place the molds in the freezer for 2 hours to set.
5. Serve.

Nutritional Values:
Calories 201
Total Fat 8.9 g
Saturated Fat 4.5 g
Cholesterol 57 mg
Sodium 340 mg
Total Carbs 24.7 g

Fiber 1.2 g
Sugar 1.3 g
Protein 15.3 g

464. Tangerine Cake

Preparation time: 10 minutes
Cooking time: 20 minutes
Servings: 8
Ingredients:

- ¾ cup coconut sugar
- 2 cups whole wheat flour
- ¼ cup olive oil
- ½ cup almond milk
- 1 teaspoon cider vinegar
- ½ teaspoon vanilla extract
- Juice and zest of 2 lemons
- Juice and zest of 1 tangerine

Directions:
1. In a bowl, mix flour with sugar and stir.
2. In another bowl, mix oil with milk, vinegar, vanilla extract, lemon juice and zest, tangerine zest and flour, whisk very well, pour this into a cake pan that fits your air fryer, introduce in the fryer and Cooking Time: at 360 degrees F for 20 minutes.
3. Serve right away.
4. Enjoy!

Nutrition: calories 210, fat 1, fiber 1, carbs 6, protein 4

465. Sweet Tomato Bread

Preparation time: 10 minutes
Cooking time: 30 minutes
Servings: 4
Ingredients:

- 1 and ½ cups whole wheat flour
- 1 teaspoon cinnamon powder
- 1 teaspoon baking powder
- 1 teaspoon baking soda

- ¾ cup maple syrup
- 1 cup tomatoes, chopped
- ½ cup olive oil
- 2 tablespoon apple cider vinegar

Directions:

1. In a bowl, mix flour with baking powder, baking soda, cinnamon and maple syrup and stir well.
2. In another bowl, mix tomatoes with olive oil and vinegar and stir well.
3. Combine the 2 mixtures, stir well, pour into a greased loaf pan that fits your air fryer, introduce in the fryer and Cooking Time: at 360 degrees F for 30 minutes.
4. Leave the cake to cool down, slice and serve.
5. Enjoy!

Nutrition: calories 203, fat 2, fiber 1, carbs 12, protein 4

466. Lemon Squares

Preparation time: 10 minutes
Cooking time: 30 minutes
Servings: 6
Ingredients:

- 1 cup whole wheat flour
- ½ cup vegetable oil
- 1 and ¼ cups coconut sugar
- 1 medium banana
- 2 teaspoons lemon peel, grated
- 2 tablespoons lemon juice
- 2 tablespoons flax meal combined with 2 tablespoons water
- ½ teaspoon baking powder

Directions:

1. In a bowl, mix flour with ¼ cup sugar and oil, stir well, press on the bottom of a pan that fits your air fryer, introduce in the fryer and bake at 350 degrees F for 14 minutes.

2. In another bowl, mix the rest of the sugar with lemon juice, lemon peel, banana, and baking powder, stir using your mixer and spread over baked crust.
3. Bake for 15 minutes more, leave aside to cool down, cut into medium squares and serve cold.
4. Enjoy!

Nutrition: calories 140, fat 4, fiber 1, carbs 12, protein 1

467. Sweet Cashew Sticks

Preparation time: 10 minutes
Cooking time: 15 minutes
Servings: 6
Ingredients:

- 1/3 cup stevia
- ¼ cup almond meal
- 1 tablespoon almond butter
- 1 and ½ cups cashews, chopped
- 4 dates, chopped
- ¾ cup coconut, shredded
- 1 tablespoon chia seeds

Directions:

1. In a bowl, mix stevia with almond meal, almond butter, cashews, coconut, dates and chia seeds and stir well again.
2. Spread this on a lined baking sheet that fits your air fryer, press well, introduce in the fryer and Cooking Time: at 300 degrees F for 15 minutes.
3. Leave mix to cool down, cut into medium sticks and serve.
4. Enjoy!

Nutrition: calories 162, fat 4, fiber 7, carbs 5, protein 6

468. Grape Pudding

Preparation time: 10 minutes
Cooking time: 40 minutes
Servings: 6
Ingredients:

- 1 cup grapes curd
- 3 cups grapes
- 3 and ½ ounces maple syrup
- 3 tablespoons flax meal combined with 3 tablespoons water
- 2 ounces coconut butter, melted
- 3 and ½ ounces almond milk
- ½ cup almond flour
- ½ teaspoon baking powder

Directions:

1. In a bowl, mix the half of the fruit curd with the grapes stir and divide into 6 heatproof ramekins.
2. In a bowl, mix flax meal with maple syrup, melted coconut butter, the rest of the curd, baking powder, milk and flour and stir well.
3. Divide this into the ramekins as well, introduce in the fryer and Cooking Time: at 200 degrees F for 40 minutes.
4. Leave puddings to cool down and serve!
5. Enjoy!

Nutrition: calories 230, fat 22, fiber 3, carbs 17, protein 8

469. Coconut And Seeds Bars

Preparation time: 10 minutes
Cooking time: 35 minutes
Servings: 4
Ingredients:

- 1 cup coconut, shredded
- ½ cup almonds
- ½ cup pecans, chopped
- 2 tablespoons coconut sugar
- ½ cup pumpkin seeds
- ½ cup sunflower seeds
- 2 tablespoons sunflower oil
- 1 teaspoon nutmeg, ground
- 1 teaspoon pumpkin pie spice

Directions:

1. In a bowl, mix almonds and pecans with pumpkin seeds, sunflower seeds, coconut, nutmeg and pie spice and stir well.
2. Heat up a pan with the oil over medium heat, add sugar, stir well, pour this over nuts and coconut mix and stir well.
3. Spread this on a lined baking sheet that fits your air fryer, introduce in your air fryer and Cooking Time: at 300 degrees F and bake for 25 minutes.
4. Leave the mix aside to cool down, cut and serve.
5. Enjoy!

Nutrition: calories 252, fat 7, fiber 8, carbs 12, protein 7

470. Chocolate Cookies

Preparation time: 10 minutes
Cooking time: 25 minutes
Servings: 12
Ingredients:

- 1 teaspoon vanilla extract
- ½ cup coconut butter, melted
- 1 tablespoon flax meal combined with 2 tablespoons water
- 4 tablespoons coconut sugar
- 2 cups flour
- ½ cup unsweetened vegan chocolate chips

Directions:

1. In a bowl, mix flax meal with vanilla extract and sugar and stir well.

2. Add melted butter, flour and half of the chocolate chips and stir everything.
3. Transfer this to a pan that fits your air fryer, spread the rest of the chocolate chips on top, introduce in the fryer at 330 degrees F and bake for 25 minutes.
4. Slice when it's cold and serve.
5. Enjoy!

Nutrition: calories 230, fat 12, fiber 2, carbs 13, protein 5

471. Simple And Sweet Bananas

Preparation time: 10 minutes
Cooking time: 15 minutes
Servings: 4
Ingredients:

- 3 tablespoons coconut butter
- 2 tablespoons flax meal combined with 2 tablespoons water
- 8 bananas, peeled and halved
- ½ cup corn flour
- 3 tablespoons cinnamon powder
- 1 cup vegan breadcrumbs

Directions:

1. Heat up a pan with the butter over medium-high heat, add breadcrumbs, stir and Cooking Time: for 4 minutes and then transfer to a bowl.
2. Roll each banana in flour, flax meal and breadcrumbs mix.
3. Arrange bananas in your air fryer's basket, dust with cinnamon sugar and Cooking Time: at 280 degrees F for 10 minutes.
4. Transfer to plates and serve.
5. Enjoy!

Nutrition: calories 214, fat 1, fiber 4, carbs 12, protein 4

472. Coffee Pudding

Preparation time: 10 minutes
Cooking time: 10 minutes
Servings: 4
Ingredients:

- 4 ounces coconut butter
- 4 ounces dark vegan chocolate, chopped
- Juice of ½ orange
- 1 teaspoon baking powder
- 2 ounces whole wheat flour
- ½ teaspoon instant coffee
- 2 tablespoons flax meal combined with 2 tablespoons water
- 2 ounces coconut sugar

Directions:

1. Heat up a pan with the coconut butter over medium heat, add chocolate and orange juice, stir well and take off heat.
2. In a bowl, mix sugar with instant coffee and flax meal, beat using your mixer, add chocolate mix, flour, salt and baking powder and stir well.
3. Pour this into a greased pan, introduce in your air fryer, Cooking Time: at 360 degrees F for 10 minutes, divide between plates and serve.
4. Enjoy!

Nutrition: calories 189, fat 6, fiber 4, carbs 14, protein 3

473. Almond And Vanilla Cake

Preparation time: 10 minutes
Cooking time: 30 minutes
Servings: 8
Ingredients:

- 1 and ½ cup stevia
- 1 cup flour
- ¼ cup cocoa powder+ 2 tablespoons

- ½ cup chocolate almond milk
- 2 teaspoons baking powder
- 2 tablespoons canola oil
- 1 teaspoon vanilla extract
- 1 and ½ cups hot water
- Cooking spray

Directions:

1. In a bowl, mix flour with 2 tablespoons cocoa, baking powder, almond milk, oil and vanilla extract, whisk well and spread on the bottom of a cake pan greased with cooking spray.
2. In a separate bowl, mix stevia with the rest of the cocoa and the water, whisk well and spread over the batter in the pan.
3. Introduce in the fryer and Cooking Time: at 350 degrees F for 30 minutes.
4. Leave the cake to cool down, slice and serve.
5. Enjoy!

Nutrition: calories 250, fat 4, fiber 3, carbs 10, protein 2

474. Blueberry Cake

Preparation time: 10 minutes
Cooking time: 30 minutes
Servings: 6
Ingredients:

- ½ cup whole wheat flour
- ¼ teaspoon baking powder
- ¼ teaspoon stevia
- ¼ cup blueberries
- 1/3 cup almond milk
- 1 teaspoon olive oil
- 1 teaspoon flaxseed, ground
- ½ teaspoon lemon zest, grated
- ¼ teaspoon vanilla extract
- ¼ teaspoon lemon extract

- Cooking spray

Directions:

1. In a bowl, mix flour with baking powder, stevia, blueberries, milk, oil, flaxseeds, lemon zest, vanilla extract and lemon extract and whisk well.
2. Spray a cake pan with cooking spray, line it with parchment paper, pour cake batter, introduce in the fryer and Cooking Time: at 350 degrees F for 30 minutes.
3. Leave the cake to cool down, slice and serve.
4. Enjoy!

Nutrition: calories 210, fat 4, fiber 4, carbs 10, protein 4

475. Peach Cobbler

Preparation time: 10 minutes
Cooking time: 30 minutes
Servings: 4
Ingredients:

- 4 cups peaches, peeled and sliced
- ¼ cup coconut sugar
- ½ teaspoon cinnamon powder
- 1 and ½ cups vegan crackers, crushed
- ¼ cup stevia
- ¼ teaspoon nutmeg, ground
- ½ cup almond milk
- 1 teaspoon vanilla extract
- Cooking spray

Directions:

1. In a bowl, mix peaches with coconut sugar and cinnamon and stir.
2. In a separate bowl, mix crackers with stevia, nutmeg, almond milk and vanilla extract and stir.
3. Spray a pie pan that fits your air fryer with cooking spray and spread peaches on the bottom.
4. Add crackers mix, spread, introduce

into the fryer and Cooking Time: at 350 degrees F for 30 minutes

5. Divide the cobbler between plates and serve.
6. Enjoy!

Nutrition: calories 201, fat 4, fiber 4, carbs 7, protein 3

476. Easy Pears Dessert

Preparation time: 10 minutes
Cooking time: 25 minutes
Servings: 12
Ingredients:

- 6 big pears, cored and chopped
- ½ cup raisins
- 1 teaspoon ginger powder
- ¼ cup coconut sugar
- 1 teaspoon lemon zest, grated

Directions:

1. In a pan that fits your air fryer, mix pears with raisins, ginger, sugar and lemon zest, stir, introduce in the fryer and Cooking Time: at 350 degrees F for 25 minutes.
2. Divide into bowls and serve cold.
3. Enjoy!

Nutrition: calories 200, fat 3, fiber 4, carbs 6, protein 6

477. Sweet Strawberry Mix

Preparation time: 10 minutes
Cooking time: 20 minutes
Servings: 10
Ingredients:

- 2 tablespoons lemon juice
- 2 pounds strawberries
- 4 cups coconut sugar
- 1 teaspoon cinnamon powder
- 1 teaspoon vanilla extract

Directions:

1. In a pan that fits your air fryer, mix

strawberries with coconut sugar, lemon juice, cinnamon and vanilla, stir gently, introduce in the fryer and Cooking Time: at 350 degrees F for 20 minutes

2. Divide into bowls and serve cold.
3. Enjoy!

Nutrition: calories 140, fat 0, fiber 1, carbs 5, protein 2

478. Sweet Bananas And Sauce

Preparation time: 10 minutes
Cooking time: 20 minutes
Servings: 4
Ingredients:

- Juice of ½ lemon
- 3 tablespoons agave nectar
- 1 tablespoon coconut oil
- 4 bananas, peeled and sliced diagonally
- ½ teaspoon cardamom seeds

Directions:

1. Arrange bananas in a pan that fits your air fryer, add agave nectar, lemon juice, oil and cardamom, introduce in the fryer and Cooking Time: at 360 degrees F for 20 minutes
2. Divide bananas and sauce between plates and serve.
3. Enjoy!

Nutrition: calories 210, fat 1, fiber 2, carbs 8, protein 3

479. Orange Cake

Preparation time: 10 minutes
Cooking time: 30 minutes
Servings: 4
Ingredients:

- Cooking spray
- 1 teaspoon baking powder
- 1 cup almond flour
- 1 cup coconut sugar

- ½ teaspoon cinnamon powder
- 3 tablespoons coconut oil, melted
- ½ cup almond milk
- ½ cup pecans, chopped
- ¾ cup water
- ½ cup raisins
- ½ cup orange peel, grated
- ¾ cup orange juice

Directions:
1. In a bowl, mix flour with half of the sugar, baking powder, cinnamon, 2 tablespoons oil, milk, pecans and raisins, stir and pour this in a greased cake pan that fits your air fryer.
2. Heat up a small pan over medium heat, add water, orange juice, orange peel, the rest of the oil and the rest of the sugar, stir, bring to a boil, pour over the mix from the pan, introduce in the fryer and Cooking Time: at 330 degrees F for 30 minutes.
3. Serve cold.
4. Enjoy!

Nutrition: calories 282, fat 3, fiber 1, carbs 4, protein 3

480. Stuffed Apples

Preparation time: 10 minutes
Cooking time: 25 minutes
Servings: 5
Ingredients:
- 5 apples, tops cut off and cored
- 5 figs
- 1/3 cup coconut sugar
- ¼ cup pecans, chopped
- 2 teaspoons lemon zest, grated
- ½ teaspoon cinnamon powder
- 1 tablespoon lemon juice
- 1 tablespoon coconut oil

Directions:
1. In a bowl mix figs, coconut sugar, pecans, lemon zest, cinnamon, lemon juice and coconut oil and stir.
2. Stuff the apples with this mix, introduce them in your air fryer and Cooking Time: at 365 degrees F for 25 minutes.
3. Enjoy!

Nutrition: calories 200, fat 1, fiber 2, carbs 6, protein 3

481. Apples And Mandarin Sauce

Preparation time: 10 minutes
Cooking time: 20 minutes
Servings: 4
Ingredients:
- 4 apples, cored, peeled and cored
- 2 cups mandarin juice
- ¼ cup maple syrup
- 2 teaspoons cinnamon powder
- 1 tablespoon ginger, grated

Directions:
1. In a pan that fits your air fryer, mix apples with mandarin juice, maple syrup, cinnamon and ginger, introduce in the fryer and Cooking Time: at 365 degrees F for 20 minutes
2. Divide apples mix between plates and serve warm.
3. Enjoy!

Nutrition: calories 170, fat 1, fiber 2, carbs 6, protein 4

482. Almond Cookies

Preparation time: 10 minutes
Cooking time: 30 minutes
Servings: 12
Ingredients:
- 1 tablespoon flaxseed mixed with 2 tablespoons water

- ¼ cup coconut oil, melted
- 1 cup coconut sugar
- ½ teaspoon vanilla extract
- 1 teaspoon baking powder
- 1 and ½ cups almond meal
- ½ cup almonds, chopped

Directions:
1. In a bowl, mix oil with sugar, vanilla extract and flax meal and whisk.
2. Add baking powder, almond meal and almonds and stir well.
3. Spread cookie mix on a lined baking sheet, introduce in your air fryer and Cooking Time: at 340 degrees F for 30 minutes.
4. Leave cookie sheet to cool down, cut into medium pieces and serve.
5. Enjoy!

Nutrition: calories 210, fat 2, fiber 1, carbs 7, protein 6

483. Easy Pumpkin Cake

Preparation time: 10 minutes
Cooking time: 40 minutes
Servings: 10
Ingredients:
- 1 and ½ teaspoons baking powder
- Cooking spray
- 1 cup pumpkin puree
- 2 cups almond flour
- ½ teaspoon baking soda
- 1 and ½ teaspoons cinnamon, ground
- ¼ teaspoon ginger, ground
- 1 tablespoon coconut oil, melted
- 1 tablespoon flaxseed mixed with 2 tablespoons water
- 1 tablespoon vanilla extract
- 1/3 cup maple syrup
- 1 teaspoon lemon juice

Directions:

1. In a bowl, flour with baking powder, baking soda, cinnamon and ginger and stir.
2. Add flaxseed, coconut oil, vanilla, pumpkin puree, maple syrup and lemon juice, stir and pour into a greased cake pan.
3. Introduce in your air fryer, Cooking Time: at 330 degrees F for 40 minutes, leave aside to cool down, slice and serve.
4. Enjoy!

Nutrition: calories 202, fat 3, fiber 2, carbs 6, protein 1

484. Sweet Potato Mix

Preparation time: 10 minutes
Cooking time: 30 minutes
Servings: 8
Ingredients:
- 1 cup water
- 1 tablespoon lemon peel, grated
- ½ cup coconut sugar
- 3 sweet potatoes peeled and sliced
- ¼ cup cashew butter
- ¼ cup maple syrup
- 1 cup pecans, chopped

Directions:
1. In a pan that fits your air fryer, mix water with lemon peel, coconut sugar, potatoes, cashew butter, maple syrup and pecans, stir, introduce in the fryer and Cooking Time: at 350 degrees F for 30 minutes
2. Divide sweet potato pudding into bowls and serve cold.
3. Enjoy!

Nutrition: calories 210, fat 4, fiber 3, carbs 10, protein 4

485. Summer Day Brownies

Preparation Time: 30 Minutes
Servings: 12
Ingredients:

- 1 cup unsweetened cocoa powder
- 1 cup whole wheat pastry flour
- 1/2 cup packed brown sugar
- 1 cup nondairy milk
- 1 teaspoon vanilla extract
- 1/4 teaspoon salt
- 1/2 cup nondairy butter
- 1/2 teaspoon baking powder
- 2 tablespoons ground flaxseed
- 2 tablespoons warm water
- Powdered sugar, for serving

Directions:

1. Mix the flaxseed with the warm water and set aside.
2. Mix together all the dry ingredients in a separate bowl.
3. In a third bowl, beat together the butter and brown sugar. Stir in the flaxseed, vanilla, and milk before stirring in the dry ingredients a little bit at a time.
4. Place a cup of water in the bottom of the instant pot, and then place a rack on top.
5. Spray a baking dish or springform pan small enough to fit in your instant pot with nonstick spray.
6. Pour the brownie batter into the greased pan and lightly cover it with foil before lowering it onto the rack.
7. Seal the lid and Cooking Time: on high for 20 minutes, quick releasing the pressure when it is finished. Dust with powdered sugar.

486. Cranberry Cheesecake

Preparation Time: 35 Minutes
Servings: 8
Ingredients:

- 2 lbs soy yogurt
- 2 cups of sugar
- 4 tbsp flaxseed mixed with ¾ cup hot water
- 2 tsp lemon zest
- 1 tsp lemon extract
- ½ tsp salt
- 1 pie crust, dairy-free

For Topping:

- 7 oz dried cranberries
- 2 tbsp cranberry jam
- 2 tsp lemon zest
- 1 tsp vanilla sugar
- 1 tsp cranberry extract
- ¾ cup lukewarm water

Directions:

1. Preheat the oven to 350 degrees. In a large bowl, combine soy yogurt, sugar, flaxseed mixture, lemon zest, lemon extract, and salt. Using an electric mixer, beat well on low until combined.
2. Grease a medium-sized springform pan with some oil. Place crust in it and pour in the filling. Flatten the surface with a spatula. Leave in the refrigerator for about 30 minutes.
3. Meanwhile, prepare the topping. Combine cranberries with cranberry jam, lemon zest, vanilla sugar, cranberry extract, and water in a small pan. Bring it to a boil and simmer for 15 minutes over medium-low heat. You can add one teaspoon of cornstarch, but this is optional.
4. Fill your instant pot with ½ inch of

water and position the trivet in the bottom. Set the cheesecake on the trivet and top with cranberries. Cover the stainless steel insert with a triple layer of paper towels and close the lid. Plug in your instant pot and set the steam release handle. Press "Manual" button and set the timer for 20 minutes.

5. Turn off the heat and let stand until the instant pot has cooled, 1 hour.

6. Run a sharp knife around the edge of your cheesecake. Refrigerate overnight.

487. Fig Spread Dessert

Preparation Time: 35 Minutes
Servings: 16
Ingredients:

- 1 cup of vegetable oil
- 1 cup of almond milk
- 1 cup of lukewarm water
- ½ cup of fig spread
- 1 ½ cup of all-purpose flour
- ½ cup of wheat groats
- ½ cup of corn flour
- 2 tsp of baking powder

Topping:

- 2 cups of brown sugar
- 2 cups of water
- ½ cup of fig spread

Directions:

1. First, you will have to prepare the topping because it has to chill well before using it. Place sugar, fig spread, and water in a heavy-bottomed pot. Bring it to a boil over a medium-high heat and Cooking Time: for 5 minutes, stirring constantly. Remove from the heat and cool well.

2. In another pot, combine oil with lukewarm water, almond milk, and fig spread. Bring it to a boil and then add flour, wheat groats, corn flour, and baking powder. Give it a good stir and mix well. Continue to Cooking Time: for 3-4 minutes. Chill well and form the dough.

3. Using your hands, shape 2-inches thick balls. This mixture should give you about 16 balls, depending on the size you want. Gently flatten the surface and transfer to a lightly greased stainless steel insert of your instant pot. Press "Manual" button and set the steam release handle. Set the timer for 10 minutes.

4. When done, press "Cancel" button and turn off your pot. Perform a quick release and open the pot. Gently remove the fig spread and pour the cold topping over them. Set aside to cool completely.

5. Refrigerate for one hour and serve.

488. Crème Brulée

Preparation Time: 11 Minutes
Servings: 4
Ingredients:

- 3 cups of coconut cream
- 3 tbsp flaxseed mixed with ½ cup hot water
- 1 cup of sugar plus 4 tbsp for topping
- 1 vanilla bean, split lengthwise
- ¼ tsp of salt

Directions:

1. In a large bowl, combine coconut cream with flaxseed mixture. Beat well with an electric mixer on high.

2. Using a sharp knife, scrape the seed out of your vanilla bean and add them to your cream mixture. I like to use the remaining of my vanilla bean. Finely chop it and add to the mixture.

This, however, is optional. You can also add one teaspoon of pure vanilla extract for some extra flavor.

3. Now, whisk in the salt and beat well again. Pour the mixture into four standard-sized ramekins. Set aside.

4. Take 4 x 12" long pieces of aluminum foil and roll them up. You want to get snake-shaped pieces of the aluminum foil. Curl each piece into a circle, pinching the ends together. Place in the bottom of the stainless steel insert of your instant pot.

5. Place each ramekin on aluminum circle and pour enough boiling water to reach up to about 1/3 of the way. Close the cooker's lid and set the steam release handle. Press "Manual" button and set the timer to 6 minutes. Cooking Time: on high pressure.

6. When done, release the steam pressure naturally for about 10 minutes, and then perform a quick release for any remaining steam.

7. Carefully remove the ramekins from the instant pot and add one tablespoon of sugar in each ramekin. Burn evenly with a culinary torch until brown.

8. Chill well and serve.

489. Chocolate Cake

Preparation Time: 45 Minutes
Servings: 12
Ingredients:

- 3 cups of soy yogurt
- 3 cups of all-purpose flour
- 2 cups of granulated sugar
- 1 cup of oil
- 2 tsp of baking soda
- 3 tbsp of cocoa, unsweetened

For the glaze:

- 7 oz dark chocolate
- 10 tbsp of sugar
- 10 tbsp of almond milk
- 5 oz almond butter, unsalted

Directions:

1. In a large bowl, combine soy yogurt, flour, sugar, oil, baking soda, and cocoa. Beat well with an electric mixer on high.

2. Transfer the mixture to a large springform pan. Wrap the pan in foil and place in your instant pot. Seal the lid and set the steam release handle. Press the "Manual" button and set the timer to 30 minutes.

3. When you hear the cooker's end signal, perform the quick release and open it. Gently remove the springform pan and unwrap. Chill well.

4. Meanwhile, melt the chocolate in a microwave. Transfer to a medium-sized bowl and whisk in almond butter, almond milk, and sugar. Beat well with an electric mixer and pour the mixture over your cake.

5. Refrigerate for at least two hours before serving.

490. Crème Caramel

Preparation Time: 30 Minutes
Servings: 4
Ingredients:

- ½ cup of granulated sugar, divided in half
- ½ cup of water
- 3 tbsp flaxseed, mixed with ½ cup hot water
- ½ tsp of vanilla extract
- ½ cup of almond milk
- 5 oz coconut cream, whipped

Directions:

1. Plug in your instant pot and press "Sautee" button.
2. In a stainless steel insert, combine ¼ cup of granulated sugar with water. Gently simmer, stirring constantly, until sugar dissolves evenly and turns into nice golden caramel. Press "Cancel" button and remove the steel insert. Set aside for 2-3 minutes, until bubbles disappear. Pour into ramekins and set aside.
3. Clean your steel insert and put it back in your instant pot.
4. Now, combine almond milk with whipped coconut cream and vanilla extract. Press "Sautee" button again and Cooking Time: for about 5 minutes, or until small bubbles form. Press the "Cancel" button and remove from the cooker.
5. Using an electric mixer, whisk the flaxseed mixture and remaining sugar. Gradually add the cream mixture and whisk until well combined. Now, pour the mixture into small ovenproof bowls and set aside.
6. Take a fitting springform pan and place ramekins in it. Fit the pan into your instant pot and pour enough water in the springform pan to reach half of the bowls. Cover the pan with a piece of foil and close the lid.
7. Press the "Manual" button and set the timer for 15 minutes. When you hear the cooker's end signal, perform a quick release and remove the lid. Crème caramel should be nice and set. If you're not sure, insert a toothpick in the middle. It will come out clean.
8. Remove the ramekins from your cooker and cool completely at a room temperature. Be careful not to refrigerate until completely chilled. Otherwise, the crème will have cracks

and it will change its structure.

491. Lemon Dessert

Preparation Time: 45 Minutes
Servings: 10
Ingredients:
- 2 cups sugar
- 2 cups vegetable oil
- ½ cup all-purpose flour
- 1 tbsp dairy-free egg replacer
- 1 tsp baking powder

Lemon topping:
- 4 cups sugar
- 5 cups water
- 1 cup freshly squeezed lemon juice
- 1 tbsp lemon zest
- 1 whole lemon, sliced

Directions:
1. In a large bowl, combine egg replacer with sugar, oil, and baking powder. Gradually add flour until the mixture is thick and slightly sticky. Using your hands, shape the balls and flatten them to half-inch thick.
2. Place in a fitting springform pan and plug in your instant pot. Pour two cups of water in a stainless steel insert and gently place the springform pan. Cover the springform with foil and seal the lid. Set the steam release handle and press the "Manual" button. Set the timer for 20 minutes.
3. After you hear the cooker's end signal, perform a quick release and open. Gently remove the springform and foil. Cool to a room temperature.
4. Now, add the remaining sugar, water, lemon juice, lemon zest, and lemon slices in your instant pot. Press the "Sautee" button and gently simmer until the sugar dissolves. Press "Cancel" button and remove the

lemon mixture.

5. Pour the hot topping over chilled dessert and set aside, allowing it to soak the lemon dressing.

492. Simple Fig Dessert

Preparation Time: 30 Minutes
Servings: 4
Ingredients:

- 2 lbs fresh figs
- 1 lb sugar
- 2 tbsp lemon zest
- 1 tsp ground nutmeg
- 10 cups water

Directions:

1. Rinse well figs and drain in a large colander.
2. Plug in your instant pot and press the "Sautee" button. Add figs, sugar, water, nutmeg, and lemon zest. Give it a good stir and cook, stirring occasionally, until half of the water evaporates.
3. Optionally, you can add ½ cup of freshly squeezed lemon or lime juice to reduce the sweet taste.
4. Press the "Cancel" button and transfer figs with the remaining liquid into glass jars, without lids. Cool to a room temperature and close the lids. Refrigerate overnight before use.

493. Sweet Pumpkin Pudding

Preparation Time: 30 Minutes
Servings: 10
Ingredients:

- 2 lbs fresh pumpkin, chopped
- 1 cup brown sugar
- 2 tbsp pumpkin juice
- 4 tbsp cornstarch
- 2 tbsp lemon zest
- 1 tsp ground nutmeg
- 10 cups water

Directions:

1. Peel and prepare the pumpkin. Scrape out seeds and chop into bite-sized pieces.
2. Plug in your instant pot and place pumpkin in the stainless steel insert. In another bowl, combine sugar with pumpkin juice. Mix well until sugar dissolves completely. Now, pour the mixture into the cooker and stir in one cup of cornstarch. Add cinnamon, cloves, and water. Give it a good stir.
3. Close the lid and press "Manual" button. Set the timer for 10 minutes.
4. When you hear the cooker's signal, perform a quick release of the pressure. Open the cooker and pour the pudding into 4 serving bowls. Cool to a room temperature and then transfer to refrigerator.

494. Chill overnight.

Wild Berries Pancakes
Preparation Time: 20 Minutes
Servings: 3
Ingredients:

- 1 cup buckwheat flour
- 2 tsp baking powder
- 1 ¼ cup almond milk
- 1 tbsp flaxseed mixed with 3 tbsp of hot water
- ½ tsp salt
- 1 tsp vanilla sugar
- 1 tsp strawberry extract
- 1 cup coconut cream
- 1 cup fresh wild berries

Directions:

1. In a medium-sized mixing bowl, combine almond milk and flaxseed

mixture. Beat well with a whisking attachment on high – until foamy. Gradually, add flour and continue to beat until combined.

2. Now, add baking powder, salt, and vanilla sugar. Continue to beat on high for 3 more minutes.

3. Plug in your instant pot and grease the stainless steel insert with some oil. Spoon 2-3 tablespoons of batter into the pot. Close the lid and set to low pressure. Press "Manual" button and set the timer for 5 minutes. Perform a quick release and repeat the process with the remaining batter.

4. Top each pancake with one tablespoon of coconut cream and wild berries. Sprinkle with strawberry extract and serve immediately.

495. Marble Bread

Preparation Time: 35 Minutes
Servings: 6
Ingredients:

- 1 cup all-purpose flour
- 1 ½ tsp baking powder
- 1 tbsp powdered stevia
- ½ tsp salt
- 1 tsp cherry extract, sugar-free
- 3 tbsp almond butter, softened
- 3 tbsp flaxseed, mixed with ½ cup hot water
- ¼ cup cocoa powder, sugar-free
- ¼ cup vegan sour cream

Directions:

1. Combine all dry ingredients except cocoa in a large mixing bowl. Mix well to combine and then add the flaxseed mixture. Beat well with a dough hook attachment for one minute. Now, add vegan sour cream, almond butter, and cherry extract. Continue to beat for 3

more minutes.

2. Divide the mixture in half and add cocoa powder in one-half of the mixture. Pour the light batter into the stainless steel insert of your instant pot. Drizzle with cocoa dough to create a nice marble pattern.

3. Close the lid and adjust the steam release handle. Press "Manual" button and set the timer for 20 minutes. Cooking Time: on low pressure.

4. When done, press "Cancel" button and release the steam pressure naturally. Let it cool for a while before transfer to the serving plate.

5. Carefully remove using a large spatula and chill completely before serving.

6. Enjoy!

496. Blueberry Strudel

Preparation Time: 50 Minutes
Servings: 8
Ingredients:

- 1 cup fresh blueberries
- 1 cup fresh raspberries
- 1 tsp blueberry extract, sugar-free
- 2 cups soy yogurt
- 2 tbsp powdered stevia
- 2 tbsp almond butter, softened
- ¼ cup cornstarch
- 2 puff pastry sheets, dairy-free
- ¼ tsp salt

Directions:

1. Place the blueberries along with stevia, cornstarch and salt in a food processor. Pulse until smooth and transfer to a heavy-bottomed pot. Add one cup of water and bring it to a boil. Briefly Cooking Time: for 3 minutes, stirring constantly. Remove from the heat and set aside to cool completely.

2. In a medium-sized bowl, combine soy

yogurt with blueberry extract- mix until completely smooth and set aside.

3. Unfold the pastry and cut each sheet into –inch x 7-inch pieces. Place approximately two tablespoons of blueberry mixture at the middle of each pastry. Fold the sheets and cut the surface with a sharp knife. Gently place each strudel into the stainless steel insert of your instant pot.

4. Plug in the instant pot and press "Manual" button. Set the timer for 25 minutes and Cooking Time: on low pressure.

5. When done, press "Cancel" button and release the steam naturally.

6. Let it chill for 10 minutes. Carefully transfer the strudels to a serving plate using a large spatula.

497. Vanilla Pancakes

Preparation Time: 37 Minutes
Servings: 6
Ingredients:

- 2 medium-sized bananas, mashed
- 1 ¼ cup almond milk
- 1 tbsp vegan egg replacer
- 1 ½ cup rolled oats
- 1 ½ tsp baking powder
- 1 tsp vanilla extract
- 2 tsp coconut oil
- 1 tbsp agave nectar
- ¼ tsp salt
- Non-fat cooking spray

Directions:

1. Combine all ingredients in a blender and pulse until completely smooth batter. Set aside.

2. Plug in your instant pot and grease the stainless steel insert with some cooking spray. Add about ¼ cup of the batter and close the lid. Press

"Manual" button and Cooking Time: for 5 minutes on low pressure.

3. Repeat the process with the remaining batter.

4. Serve immediately.

498. Apple Pie Cups With Cranberries

Preparation Time: 120 Minutes
Servings: 6
Ingredients:
For the crust:

- 2 cups all-purpose flour
- ¾ tsp salt
- ¾ cup almond butter, softened
- 1 tbsp sugar
- ½ cup ice water

For the filling:

- 1 medium-sized Alkmene apple
- ½ fresh peach
- ½ cup blackberries
- ¼ cup cranberries
- 2 tbsp all-purpose flour
- 1 tbsp sugar
- ½ tsp cinnamon

Directions:

1. Place all the crust ingredients in a food processor and pulse until dough is crumbly, but holds together when squeezed. Remove from the food processor and place on a lightly floured work surface. Divide in 4 equal pieces and wrap in plastic foil. Refrigerate for one hour.

2. Meanwhile, place all filling ingredients in a medium-sized bowl. Toss to combine and set aside.

3. Roll each piece into 6-inch round discs. Add two tablespoons of the apple mixture at the center of each disc and wrap to form small bowls. Gently transfer to the stainless steel insert of your instant pot and sprinkle

with cooking spray.

4. Plug in your instant pot and press "Manual" button. Set the timer for 25 minutes and adjust the steam release handle. Cooking Time: on low pressure.
5. When done, press "Cancel" button and release the steam naturally. Carefully transfer cups to the serving plate and enjoy!

499. Blueberry Peach Pie

Preparation Time: 75 Minutes
Servings: 6
Ingredients:

- 1 cup fresh blueberries
- 1 medium-sized peach, sliced
- 1 cup all-purpose flour
- 2 tbsp flaxseed, mixed with ¼ cup of hot water
- 1 tsp baking powder
- ½ tsp salt
- ¼ cup almond butter, softened
- ¼ cup powdered stevia
- ¼ tsp vanilla extract
- 2 tsp freshly squeezed lemon juice

Directions:

1. In a medium-sized bowl, combine flour, baking powder, and salt. Mix well and set aside.
2. In a separate bowl, combine flaxseed mixture and stevia powder. Using a hand mixer with a whisking attachment, beat well on high for 2 minutes, or until light and fluffy.
3. Place the flour mixture in a large mixing bowl. Add almond butter, vanilla extract, and lemon juice. Gradually add the flaxseed mixture, beating constantly. Continue to beat for 3-5 minutes.
4. Place the flour mixture into the stainless steel insert of your instant pot. Spread the batter evenly with a

kitchen spatula. Arrange the fruit on top and close the lid. Adjust the steam release handle and press "Manual" button. Set the timer for 30 minutes. Cooking Time: on low pressure.
5. When done, press "Cancel" button and release the steam naturally. Remove from the pot and chill completely before serving.

500. Vanilla Ice Cream

Ingredients

- 1 (13.5-ounce can coconut milk
- 1½ cups almond or soy milk
- ¾ cup agave
- 3 tablespoons olive oil
- 1 teaspoon pure vanilla extract
- ⅛ teaspoon salt
- ¾ teaspoon xanthan gum

Directions:

Process coconut milk, almond milk, agave, oil, vanilla extract, salt, and xanthan gum in a blender. Chill in the refrigerator for 3 hours. Once the ice cream base is chilled, prepare in an ice-cream maker per manufacturer's instructions.

CONCLUSION

Thanks for making to the end! I hope you enjoy all the recipes herein. If dieting seems very important to you and you need to do it right, then it is recommended that you visit a professional such as a nutritionist or dietitian to discuss your dieting plan and optimizing it for the better.

No matter how much you want to lose weight, it is not advised that you decrease your calorie intake to an unhealthy level. Losing weight does not mean that you stop eating. It is done by carefully planning meals.

A plant-based diet is very easy once you get into it. At first, you will start to face a lot of difficulties, but if you start slowly, then you can face all the barriers and achieve your goal

Lightning Source UK Ltd.
Milton Keynes UK
UKHW030629080321
379980UK00010B/1557